Mark Findlay • Christopher Isles

Clinical Companion in Nephrology

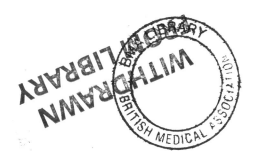

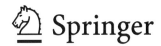 Springer

Mark Findlay
Institute of Cardiovascular and Medical
Sciences
University of Glasgow
Glasgow
UK

Christopher Isles
Dumfries and Galloway Royal Infirmary
Dumfries
UK

ISBN 978-3-319-14867-0   ISBN 978-3-319-14868-7   (eBook)
DOI 10.1007/978-3-319-14868-7

Library of Congress Control Number: 2015938307

Springer Cham Heidelberg New York Dordrecht London

Printed on acid-free paper

Springer International Publishing AG Switzerland is part of Springer Science+Business Media
(www.springer.com)

Clinical Companion in Nephrology

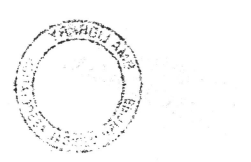

Preface

We have written this clinical companion for medical students and junior doctors who have told us over the years that renal medicine is 'too difficult' and not always well covered in textbooks. We suspect this may be a consequence of a tendency to concentrate on mechanisms as a prerequisite for understanding disease and we have made a conscious decision to avoid this approach. Renal physiology and pathophysiology are undoubtedly interesting but they are also complex and a *detailed* knowledge of what happens inside the renal tubule is probably not necessary to assess, investigate and manage a patient with acute kidney injury or chronic kidney disease.

We have also made a conscious decision to divide the text into bite size chunks using a Q and A format. We have done this partly because we have found this approach works when teaching and partly because there is so much more to learn than there was 20–30 years ago. With this approach in mind we have divided our material into six sections. We start with the physiology that it helps to know and go on to assess GFR, proteinuria and haematuria. We include a section on electrolyte and acid-base disorders next as nephrologists are frequently asked for help in these areas. We devote considerable space to AKI and CKD because these topics are most likely to be encountered by general medical trainees. We then describe a miscellaneous group of renal topics including urinary tract infection and renal stones before tackling renal replacement therapy in a way that we hope will make clearer to non-nephrologists exactly what goes on inside dialysis and transplant units. We conclude with a series of appendices. We have always taught students that there are some things they need to know and some things they need to look up. The appendices are where medical students and junior doctors will find material they don't always need to carry in their heads.

We are grateful to a number of colleagues who have reviewed chapters for us, helped with illustrations or provided us with slides. In particular we would like to thank Alison Almond, Zeyad Bayaty, Lynn Carson, Louise Clark, Fiona Gardiner, Fiona Green, David Kipgen, Thalakunte Muniraju, Calum Murray, Sue Robertson, Subrata Saha, Ranjit Thomas, Abdul Wahab and Wayne Wrathall. We also acknowledge many other colleagues, especially John Firth and Roger Greenwood, whose lectures have stimulated us to consider different ways of approaching and teaching a particular topic. Last but by no means least we thank our wives, Maytal and Karen, for their tolerance and patience during the many evenings we spent drafting and redrafting this book.

Glasgow, UK
Dumfries, UK

Mark Findlay
Christopher Isles

Contents

Abbreviations

1y	Primary
2y	Secondary
3y	Tertiary
AonCKD	Acute on chronic kidney disease
ABPM	Ambulatory blood pressure monitor
ACE	Angiotensin converting enzyme
ACEi	Angiotensin converting enzyme inhibitor
ACR	Albumin:creatinine ratio
ADH	Anti-diuretic hormone
ADPKD	Autosomal dominant polycystic kidney disease
AIDS	Acquired immunodeficiency syndrome
AKI	Acute kidney injury
ANA	Anti-nuclear antibody
ANCA	Anti-neutrophil cytoplasmic antibody
ANP	Atrial natriuretic peptide
Anti-GBM	Anti-glomerular basement membrane
APD	Automated peritoneal dialysis
ARB	Angiotensin II receptor blocker
ARVD	Atherosclerotic reno-vascular disease
ATN	Acute tubular necrosis
AV	Arterio-venous
BBV	Blood borne viruses
BC	Blood culture
bd	bis die (twice daily)
BJP	Bence Jones proteinuria
BP	Blood pressure
Ca	Calcium
CAPD	Continuous ambulatory peritoneal dialysis
CCB	Calcium channel blocker
CCD	Cortical collecting duct
CJD	Creutzfeldt-Jakob disease
CK	Creatine kinase
CKD	Chronic kidney disease
CM	Conservative management
CMV	Cytomegalo virus
CNI	Calcineurin inhibitor

CNS	Central nervous system
COPD	Chronic obstructive pulmonary disease
CPN	Chronic pyelonephritis
CRBSI	Catheter related blood stream infection
CRP	C-reactive protein
CT	Computed tomography
CXR	Chest X-ray
DBD	Donation following brain death
DCD	Donation following cardiac death
DCT	Distal convoluted tubule
ECF	Extra-cellular fluid
ECV	Extracellular volume
EPO	Erythropoetin
ESA	Erythropoiesis stimulating agent
ESBL	Extended-spectrum beta-lactamase
ESP	Encapsulating sclerosing perionitis
FMD	Fibro-muscular dysplasia
GFR	Glomerular filtration rate
GN	Glomerulonephritis
GPA	Granulomatous polyarteritis
GTN	Glyceryl trinitrate
Hb	Haemoglobin
HBc	Hepatitis B core
HBPM	Home blood pressure monitor
HBsAg	Hepatitis B surface antigen
HBV	Hepatitis B virus
HCV	Hepatitis C virus
HD	Haemodialysis
HELLP	Haemolysis, elevated liver enzymes, low platelets
HF	Heart failure
HIV	Human immunodeficiency
HLA	Human leukocyte antigens
HPT	Hyperparathyroidism
HR	Heart rate
HRS	Hepato-renal syndrome
HUS	Haemolytic uraemic syndrome
ICV	Intracellular volume
INR	International normalised ratio
IV	Intra-venous
IVP	Intra-venous pyelogram
K	Potassium
L	Litre
L of H	Loop of Henle
LMWH	Low molecular weight heparin
LV	Left ventricle
LVH	Left ventricular hypertrophy
MCV	Mean cell volume
MDRD	Modification of diet in renal disease

mg	Milligram
ml	Millilitres
MMF	Mycophenolate mofetil
MPA	Microscopic polyarteritis
Na	Sodium
NICE	National Institute for Health and Care Excellence
NSAID	Non-steroidal anti-inflammatory drug
OA	Osteoarthritis
Osm	Osmolality
PCP	Pneumocystis carinii pneumonia
PCR	Protein:creatinine ratio
PCT	Proximal convoluted tubule
PD	Peritoneal dialysis
PEX	Plasma Exchange
PO4	Phosphate
PTH	Parathyroid hormone
PTLD	Post-transplant lymphoproliferative disorder
qds	quarter die sumendum (four times a day)
RAAS	Renin-aldosterone-angiotensin system
RPGN	Rapidly progressive glomerulonephritis
RR	Relative risk
RRT	Renal replacement therapy
RVD	Reno-vascular disease
SC	Sub-cutaneous
SCr	Serum creatinine
(S)FLC	(Serum) free light chains
SIADH	Syndrome of inappropriate ADH
STING	Subureteral transurethral injection
TAL	Thick ascending limb (of Henle)
TCVC	Tunnelled central venous catheter
tds	ter die sumendum (three time a day)
TIPS	Transjugular intrahepatic portosystemic shunt
TLD	Thiazide-like diuretic
TSAT	Transferrin saturation
TTP	Thrombotic thrombocytopenic purpura
U&E	Urea and electrolytes
UF	Ultrafiltration
ULN	Upper limit of normal
URR	Urea reduction ratio
USS	Ultrasound scan
UTI	Urinary tract infection
vWF	von Willebrand factor
VZV	Varicella zoster virus
WCC	White cell count
WHO	World Health Organisation

Part I

Physiology and Assessment

Structure and Function of the Kidney

1

Q1 Draw and label a nephron (Fig. 1.1)

The nephron consists of a glomerulus, a proximal tubule, the loop of Henle with its thick ascending limb, the distal tubule and the cortical collecting duct. In reality, the glomerulus lies a little closer to the distal tubule than shown in our drawing, enabling the juxtaglomerular apparatus, which produces renin, to sense sodium levels in the distal tubule (see later). Healthy glomeruli filter around 100 ml of blood to produce around 1 ml of urine per minute.

Q2 List the functions of the kidney

There are four functions relating to waste, water, electrolytes and acids:
1. Excretion of metabolic waste products e.g. urea and creatinine.
2. Regulation of body water volume.
3. Regulation of electrolyte balance, particularly sodium and potassium.
4. Regulation of acid base balance.
   And four hormonal functions:
1. Mineral metabolism
2. Production of renin.

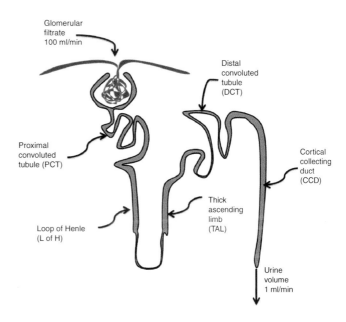

Fig. 1.1 Anatomy of a nephron

M. Findlay, C. Isles, *Clinical Companion in Nephrology*,
DOI 10.1007/978-3-319-14868-7_1, © Springer International Publishing Switzerland 2015

3. Production of erythropoietin – *see* Chap. 27
4. Role in glucose metabolism – *see* Chap. 22

We will devote the rest of this chapter to describing these functions in more detail. We do so from a clinician's rather than a physiologist's view in the belief that clinically relevant physiology is more easily remembered.

Q3   Explain how the kidney excretes urea and creatinine?

The waste products which are of most interest in monitoring excretory renal function are urea and creatinine. Both are freely filtered at the glomerulus. The tubules then re-absorb some urea (but not creatinine) and secrete some creatinine (but not urea). The body's ability to excrete waste products is determined by the glomerular filtration rate (GFR). Normal GFR is approximately 100 ml/min. The human body can tolerate a substantial loss in renal function before suffering significant ill-effects and it is not until the GFR falls below 30 ml/min that things begin to go seriously wrong (Fig. 1.2).

Q4   How do the kidneys regulate body water volume?

If our glomerular filtration rate is approximately 100 ml/min and average urinary output is only 1 ml/min (1,500 ml per day), this means that 99 ml of glomerular filtrate is reabsorbed every minute. The concentration of urine in this way is driven by a series of complex mechanisms, which we can simplify as follows:

1. The proximal convoluted tubule (PCT) and Loop of Henle reabsorb huge amounts of sodium, which creates a hyperosmolar medulla.
2. Water follows passively through the Loop of Henle in an attempt to reduce the hyperosmolarity.
3. Fine tuning of body water volume takes place in the distal convoluted tubule (DCT) and cortical collecting duct (CCD) under the influence of aldosterone and in the CCD under the influence of antidiuretic hormone.
4. The production of aldosterone and ADH is regulated by anti-natriuretic peptide (ANP) released by the atria of the heart in response to changes in central body water volume (Fig. 1.3).

For example if a patient is volume overloaded (or 'wet') the atria release ANP. ANP switches off the production of aldosterone by the adrenal cortex and of ADH by the posterior pituitary. A lack of aldosterone and ADH mean that the kidney excretes more salt and water thereby restoring normal central body volume.

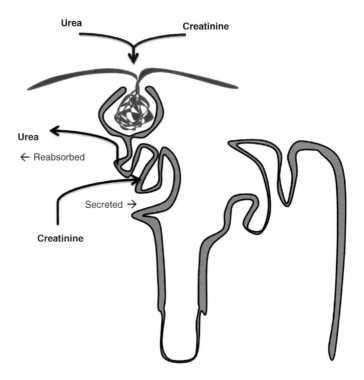

Fig. 1.2 Movement of urea and creatinine within the nephron

Fig. 1.3 Regulation of
body water

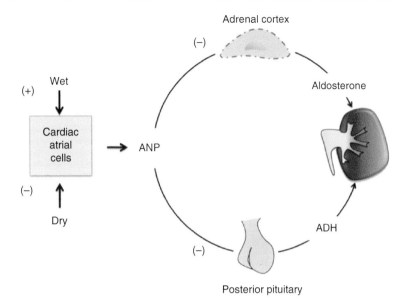

Fig. 1.4 Regulation of
sodium

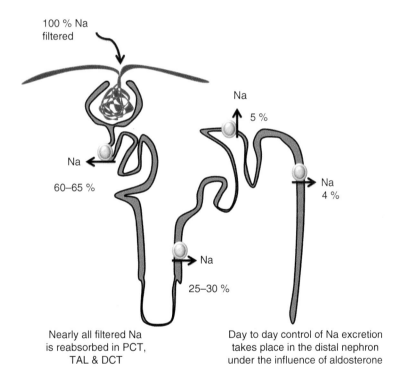

Nearly all filtered Na
is reabsorbed in PCT,
TAL & DCT

Day to day control of Na excretion
takes place in the distal nephron
under the influence of aldosterone

Q5   How do the kidneys regulate sodium?

The tubules may be thought of as having an insatiable desire to reabsorb sodium. This is an active process. Sodium is transported out of tubule and back into the body by a series of pumps in the proximal convoluted tubule (65 %), thick ascending limb of the Loop of Henle (25 %), distal convoluted tubule (5 %) and cortical collecting duct (5 %). The pumps in the distal nephron are under the influence of aldosterone (Fig. 1.4).

Q6   How do the kidneys regulate potassium?

Regulation of potassium is another critically important function of the kidney. Dietary intake is usually of the order 50–100 mmol/day. The bulk of our body's potassium is stored

Fig. 1.5 Regulation of potassium

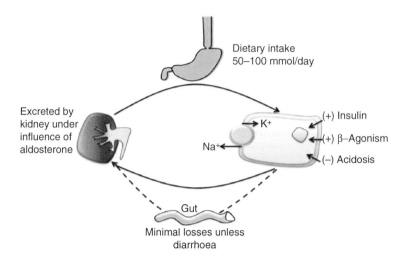

Fig. 1.6 Renal excretion of potassium

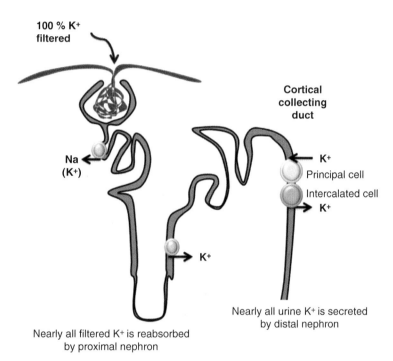

intracellularly, specifically in muscle. Potassium is actively pumped into muscle cells by a number of mechanisms (shown in Fig. 1.5), three of which we take advantage of when treating patients with hyperkalaemia (see Chap. 18).

The kidney is mainly responsible for excreting potassium from the body with the gut playing a lesser role unless the patient has diarrhoea. Nearly all filtered potassium is reabsorbed passively with sodium in the PCT (Fig. 1.6), and actively with sodium in the thick ascending limb of the Loop of Henle. Nearly all urine potassium is secreted by the principal cells of the cortical collecting duct of the distal nephron under the influence of aldosterone. The intercalated cell of the CCD is responsible for reabsorbing potassium when hypokalaemia is present.

Q7 How do the kidneys regulate acid base balance?

The kidneys play an important role in maintaining the body's hydrogen ion concentration (pH) within fairly narrow and well defined limits. Normal hydrogen ion concentration is between 35 and 45, corresponding to a pH of between 7.36 and 7.44. The kidney does this in three ways (Fig. 1.7):

1. By glomerular filtration of acids.
2. By reabsorption of bicarbonate at the proximal convoluted tubule.
3. By secretion of hydrogen ions at the cortical collecting duct.

Detailed knowledge of the regulation of acid base balance by the kidney is not necessary. Both glomerular and tubular dysfunction can lead to acidosis. Patients with advanced renal failure are acidotic mainly because they no longer filter acids. Renal tubular acidosis (RTA) occurs when the tubules fail to appropriately acidify the urine.

Q8   Describe the kidney's contribution to mineral metabolism.

The kidney plays an important role in PTH, Vitamin D, calcium and phosphate metabolism. Much of this activity is centred on maintaining a normal serum calcium. In health, low serum calcium triggers the parathyroid gland to produce PTH. This has multiple functions with one goal – raising serum calcium. This is achieved in three ways. First, PTH has a direct action on bone increasing osteoclastic activity which releases calcium into the blood stream. Second, PTH stimulates calcium reabsorption and phosphate secretion by the kidneys. Third, PTH increases the activity of the 1 alpha hydroxylase enzyme that converts inactive Vitamin D (25OHD) to its active form (1,25(OH)$_2$D). 1,25(OH)$_2$D stimulates the reabsorption of calcium from the gut. Once the serum calcium in back in the normal range, the secretion of PTH is 'switched off' by negative feedback (Fig. 1.8).

Q9   How do the kidneys regulate blood pressure?

Renin is an enzyme secreted by the juxtaglomerular apparatus (JGA) of the kidney in response to a number of stimuli, principally a fall in renal perfusion pressure and sodium depletion. The JGA lies between the glomerulus and the DCT which allows the JGA to sense the sodium concentration in the DCT. Renin converts angiotensinogen to angiotensin I which in turn is converted to angiotensin II by Angiotensin Converting Enzyme (ACE). Angiotensin II has a number of important actions both within the kidney and in the systemic circulation including a direct pressor

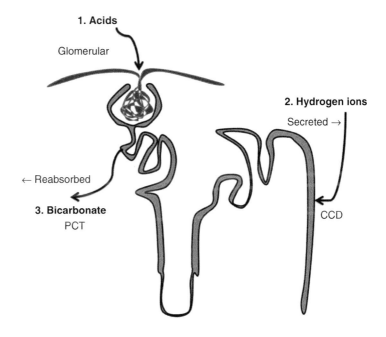

Fig. 1.7 Regulation of acid–base balance

Fig. 1.8 PTH action in
response to low serum
calcium

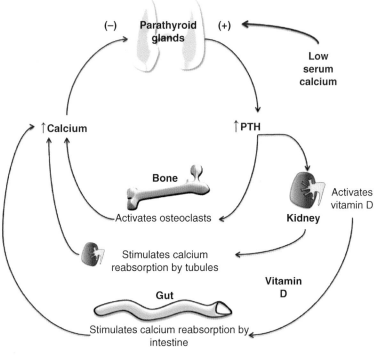

Fig. 1.9 The Renin-
Angiotensin-Aldosterone
system

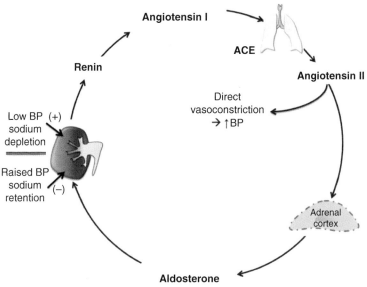

effect raising blood pressure. It also stimulates the
adrenal gland to produce aldosterone which leads
to sodium retention and potassium excretion by
the kidney, with negative feedback that then
switches off the production of renin (see Fig. 1.9).
In health, the renin angiotensin system is a mechanism for controlling blood pressure by raising
blood pressure when it is too low and lowering it
when blood pressure is too high. Increased production of renin in patients with renovascular disease is one of the mechanisms for the development
of hypertension in that disorder.

1.1   Objectives: Structure and Functions of the Kidney

After reading this chapter, you should be able to answer the following:

Q1   Draw and label a nephron

Q2   List the functions of the kidney

Q3   Explain how the kidney excretes urea and creatinine?

Q4   How do the kidneys regulate body water volume?

Q5   How do the kidneys regulate sodium balance?

Q6   How do the kidneys regulate potassium?

Q7   How do the kidneys regulate acid base balance?

Q8   Describe the kidney's contribution to mineral metabolism

Q9   How do the kidneys regulate blood pressure?

Q1 How accurate is blood urea as a measure of renal function?

When we talk about "renal function" we usually mean the glomerular filtration rate (GFR). Each kidney has around 1,000,000 nephrons and the GFR is a measure of the function of all of these in both kidneys. Urea is a nitrogenous waste product, the level of which in the blood is usually <7 mmol/l. Blood urea rises in patients with kidney injury but is an imperfect marker of GFR for the following reasons: urea generation is low in patients with chronic liver disease and malnutrition and is disproportionately increased in those who are dehydrated (because urea is reabsorbed passively with sodium and water by the proximal tubule) or those who have gastrointestinal blood loss (because urea is absorbed from the gut).

Q2 How accurate is serum creatinine as a measure of renal function?

Still imperfect but better than urea. The normal range for serum creatinine is usually given as 60–125 umol/l though all this means is that 95 % of the adult population will have a serum creatinine that lies somewhere between these two levels – serum creatinine of 125 umol/l is actually quite abnormal (see below). Creatinine is derived from creatine which is a protein found in muscle. It follows that creatinine levels will be lower in the elderly because of their lower muscle mass and higher in weight lifters. The important consequence of low muscle mass in the elderly is that elderly patients may have quite advanced renal failure with only modest elevations of their serum creatinine

Q3 What is the relation between serum creatinine & glomerular filtration rate (GFR)?

A useful rule of thumb is that every time the creatinine doubles the GFR will halve. Thus, if serum creatinine of 62.5 µmol/l and a GFR of 100 ml/min is our starting point, this means that by the time serum creatinine has gone above the upper limit of the normal range (approximately 125 µmol/l), 50 % of glomerular function has already been lost; also that when serum creatinine exceeds 500 µmol/l the GFR will have fallen below 12.5 ml/min (Fig. 2.1).

Q4 How was GFR assessed in the past?

Previously we assessed GFR by collecting urine for 24 h and measuring creatinine clearance using the formula UV/P where U = urine creatinine in µmol/l, V = volume of urine passed in ml/min and P = serum creatinine in µmol/l. This method has fallen out of favour. Not only was the collection messy and cumbersome but patients often forgot to include all the urine they passed and sometimes failed to understand that the first specimen of urine on the first day had to be discarded (Fig. 2.2)

Q5 How is GFR assessed now?

The standard method of estimating GFR now is based on the MDRD equation (so

M. Findlay, C. Isles, *Clinical Companion in Nephrology*,
DOI 10.1007/978-3-319-14868-7_2, © Springer International Publishing Switzerland 2015

Fig. 2.1 Relationship of
serum creatinine to GFR

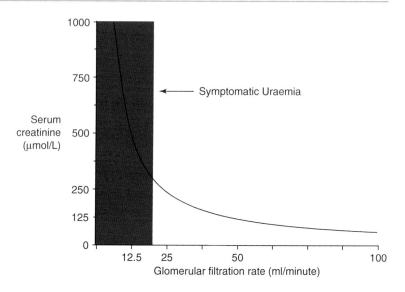

called because it was used in the study on the Modification of Diet and Renal Disease) which estimates GFR on the basis of a patient's age, serum creatinine, gender and race. All biochemistry departments in the UK now use this formula to estimate GFR. If you want to calculate eGFR on an existing creatinine result there is an easy to use calculator on the website of the Renal Association at http://egfrcalc.renal.org/

Q6 What is the Cockcroft-Gault equation?

Another equation for estimating excretory renal function. Cockcroft Gault estimates creatinine clearance (not GFR though the distinction between the two is somewhat academic) on the basis of a patients age, gender, race, serum creatinine and ideal body weight. Because Cockcroft Gault requires an estimate of ideal body weight it is not practical in everyday clinical practice but it is sometimes useful at extremes of body weight as the MDRD equation performs less well in such patients.

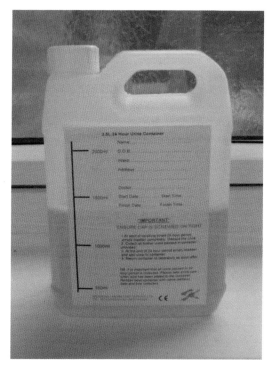

Fig. 2.2 Twenty four hour urine collection sample

Box 2.1 Changing Methods of Measuring Renal Function
Previously
• Twenty four hour urine for creatinine clearance
Nowadays
• Prediction equations for GFR e.g. MDRD, Cockcroft-Gault formula

Q7 Describe the pros and cons of estimating rather than measuring GFR

The main advantage of eGFR is that it does not require a measurement of body weight. Limitations are as follows:

- eGFR is likely to be less accurate at extremes of body type e.g. malnourished, amputees, morbidly obese.
- It underestimates GFR in Afro-Caribbeans (in whom the eGFR should be multiplied by 1.2) but works well in the UK white population and in Asians living in the UK.
- eGFR underestimates normal or near normal renal function.
- eGFR overestimates renal function in patients with advanced kidney disease particularly if they are underweight (in this circumstance, you should estimate creatinine clearance using the Cockcroft Gault equation which is based on age, gender, race, serum creatinine and body weight).
- eGFR is not valid for under 18 s or if the serum creatinine level is changing because renal function is unstable, and must not be used to estimate residual renal function in patients with acute kidney injury

Box 2.2 Accuracy of the MDRD Equation

MDRD equation is most precise when GFR is in the range 40–60 ml/min. It tends to overestimate GFR when this is low and underestimate GFR when this is greater than 60 ml/min which is the reason why most biochemistry labs simply report 'eGFR >60 ml/min' for a patient whose renal function is normal.

Q8 NICE discuss new ways of estimating GFR in their 2014 guideline. What are these?

NICE suggest measuring serum cystatin C in place of serum creatinine and using the Chronic Kidney Disease Epidemiology Collaboration (CKD-EPI) equation in place of the MDRD formula to estimate GFR when highly accurate

measures of GFR are required. Cystatin C is a low molecular weight protein that is filtered by the glomerulus, neither secreted nor reabsorbed by the renal tubules and less influenced by age, gender, race and muscle mass than creatinine. At the time of writing neither of these recommendations has found their way into routine clinical practice.

Q9 Estimating GFR has led to a new way of classifying chronic kidney disease. Discuss.

Patients may be classified by the severity of their renal failure using the MDRD equation to give an estimate of glomerular filtration rate as follows:

Box 2.3 Classification of CKD by GFR
- CKD1 – GFR >90 ml/min
- CKD2 – GFR 60–90 ml/min
- CKD3a – GFR 45–59 ml/min
- CKD3b – GFR 30–44 ml/min
- CKD4 – GFR 15–29 ml/min
- CKD5 – GFR <15 ml/min

Around 5 % of the general population have CKD3 which can be further subdivided for prognostic purposes into CKD3a which means GFR 45–59 ml/min and CKD3b which means GFR 30–44 ml/min. Patients with CKD 1 and 2 have structural abnormalities of the kidney and/or urinary abnormalities with normal renal function (eGFR >60 ml/min). The letter P is sometimes applied to indicate whether a CKD3 patient has proteinuria (arbitrarily urine PCR >100 mg/mmol). CKD4 and CKD5 are much less common, representing no more than 0.1–0.2 % of the general population.

Q10 NICE have proposed a new classification of CKD in their 2014 guideline. Discuss.

NICE have chosen to redesignate CKD1 as G1, CKD2 as G2 etc., (where G stands for GFR). They have also chosen to add an A suffix to indicate the level of proteinuria, namely A1 for urine

ACR <3 mg/mmol; A2 for urine ACR 3–30 mg/mmol: and A3 for patients with urine ACR >30 mg/mmol. Thus a patient with eGFR 50 ml/min and an ACR of 35 mg/mmol will be coded CKD G3aA3. NICE hope that this will facilitate the introduction of an international classification and risk based approach to care. It is too early to say how widely this new classification of CKD will be adopted.

Q11 Describe how severity of CKD may be related to treatment goals.

Classification of CKD by severity has the advantage that it can be used to prompt actions or treatments that are appropriate for each stage of renal failure. Thus for CKD3, the main goal of treatment is to reduce the risk of cardiovascular disease and slow the rate of progression of renal disease, wherever possible. For CKD4 the goals of treatment are all of the above and referral to a nephrologist in order to prepare for dialysis where this would be appropriate. CKD5 is the stage at which dialysis should be initiated if and when indicated.

Box 2.4 CKD Treatment Goals

CKD 1 & CKD 2

Those with normal excretory function but abnormal urine dip/renal anatomy – Monitor.

CKD 3

The "at *(further)* risk" group, who need cardiovascular disease & CKD progression prevention.

CKD 4

Refer to a nephrologist, if not already done so. Discuss whether for RRT or conservative care with patient.

CKD 5

Patients with a creatinine in the "symptomatic range". Start dialysis when indicated if RRT chosen

2.1   Objectives: Assessment of GFR

After reading this chapter you should be able to answer the following:

Q1   How accurate is blood urea as a measure of renal function?

Q2   How accurate is serum creatinine as a measure of renal function?

Q3   What is the relation between serum creatinine and glomerular filtration rate (GFR)?

Q4   How was GFR assessed in the past?

Q5   How is GFR assessed now?

Q6   What is the Cockcroft Gault equation?

Q7   Describe the pros and cons of estimating rather than measuring GFR.

Q8   NICE discuss new ways of estimating GFR in their 2014 guideline. What are these?

Q9   Estimating GFR has led to a new way of classifying chronic kidney disease. Discuss.

Q10   NICE have proposed a new classification of CKD in their 2014 guideline. Discuss.

Q11   Describe how severity of CKD may be related to treatment goals.

Further Reading

1. National Institute for Health and Care Excellence. Chronic kidney disease: early identification and management of chronic kidney disease in primary and secondary care. CG182. London: National Institute for Health and Care Excellence; 2014.

Proteinuria

Q1   What is proteinuria and how is it classified?

Proteinuria simply means the presence of protein in the urine. We all pass a small amount of protein in our urine – up to 150 mg daily. Proteinuria in excess of this may be classified as transient, postural or persistent. Transient proteinuria occurs after vigorous exercise, during febrile illnesses and in heart failure. Postural (aka orthostatic) proteinuria occurs in young adults after standing for prolonged periods. It disappears after lying down and can therefore be excluded in an early morning specimen. Postural proteinuria is completely benign. The rest of this chapter will be devoted to the discussion of persistent proteinuria, which may be further classified by severity into microalbuminuria, true proteinuria and nephrotic range proteinuria (see below).

Q2   How is proteinuria detected?

There are three methods: the urine dipstick test, the 24 h urine collection and the measurement of albumin or protein:creatinine ratio in a spot specimen. Discussion of the advantage and limitations of these tests follows.

Q3   Discuss the advantages and limitations of the dipstick test for measuring urine protein.

The dipstick test, which detects primarily albumin in the urine, is the simplest measure of proteinuria. It is a useful screening test but has a number of limitations as shown in the box:

Box 3.1 Limitations of Urine Dipstick Testing

- Insufficiently sensitive for microalbuminuria (very small amounts of albumin).
- Semi-quantitative only. Negative or trace proteinuria is rarely of clinical significance, + protein approximate to 300 mg/l which is roughly the point of transition between microalbuminuria and proteinuria. ++ protein is equivalent to 1 g/l.
- Measures urinary protein concentration rather than total urine protein passed in a day.
- Poor observer agreement if result read manually rather than by automated urine dipstick analyser.
- False negative test seen in dilute urine and when protein other than albumin e.g. Bence Jones protein is present in the urine.
- False positive tests seen in concentrated urine and in presence of haematuria.

Despite these reservations the urine dipstick test is an important and often neglected part of the initial assessment of patients with both AKI and CKD. It is surprising how often patients with AKI in particular are referred to nephrologists before their urine has been dipped for blood and protein.

M. Findlay, C. Isles, *Clinical Companion in Nephrology*,
DOI 10.1007/978-3-319-14868-7_3, © Springer International Publishing Switzerland 2015

Table 3.1 Approximations of ACR, PCR and 24 h urine collection values

	Urine ACR mg/mmol	Urine PCR mg/mmol	24 h urine protein
Normal	<3	(<15)	<150 mg
Microalbuminuria	3–30	(15–50)	150–500 mg
Proteinuria	(>30)	>50	>500 mg
Nephrotic range proteinuria	(>300)	>350	>3.5 g

Q4 What is Bence Jones proteinuria?

Bence Jones proteins (BJP) are free light chains detected in the urine of patients with myeloma and primary amyloidosis. They are identified by electrophoresis rather than by the urine dipstick test which detects albumin and not globulins. Historically the investigation of a patient with suspected myeloma has been by blood for serum electrophoresis and urine for BJP, though this is changing with the introduction of highly sensitive serum free light chain assays. Clonal production of free light chains can be detected earlier in serum than urine because of the reabsorptive capacity of the renal tubules (up to 20–30 g of free light chains can be reabsorbed daily).

Q5 Why is a 24 h urine collection for quantifying urine protein no longer recommended?

Up until recently the answer to 'how do we quantify urine protein?' would have been 'by 24 h urine collection'. This method of measuring urine protein has recently been abandoned due to a combination of inaccuracies in collection, the cumbersome nature of this process and validation of a simpler test (see below). Patients are still asked to collect their urine for twenty four hours occasionally, for example when estimating residual renal function in a patient on peritoneal dialysis. To improve accuracy the following instructions are useful.

Box 3.2 Explaining to a patient how to collect their 24 h urine
1. Wake up on the day you plan to collect it, and empty your bladder into the toilet as normal.
2. From THAT POINT ON, collect all urine passed in the container provided.

---

3. The following morning, pass the first urine of the day into the container then stop collecting.

Q6 How is urine protein quantified currently?

The answer is by sending 10 ml of urine in a white topped universal container to biochemistry requesting a urine albumin:creatinine ratio (ACR) or protein:creatinine ratio (PCR). Either the first void of the day or the next void will do. Expressing urine albumin or urine protein as a ratio with creatinine will correct for urinary concentration.

Q7 ACR or PCR?

NICE suggest urine ACR because urine ACR is more accurate than PCR at lower levels of protein output. However, when urine ACR is greater than 30 mg/mmol it is acceptable to measure urinary PCR because PCR is as accurate and considerably cheaper at higher levels of proteinuria. Urine ACR of 30 mg/mmol is roughly equivalent to urine PCR of 50 mg/mmol and to 24 h urine protein of 500 mg. which is a useful threshold for deciding whether or not a patient has true proteinuria. Another useful conversion is ACR 70 mg/mmol to PCR 100 mg/mmol and 24 h urine protein 1G. The higher the urine PCR the more likely the protein is to be glomerular in origin with PCR values greater than 200 mg/mmol nearly always indicating glomerular rather than tubular pathology. The table shows thresholds for microalbuminuria, proteinuria and nephrotic range proteinuria using the different measures of urine protein (Table 3.1).

Q8 What do you understand by the term microalbuminuria?

Literally this means the urinary excretion of very small amounts of albumin. The detection

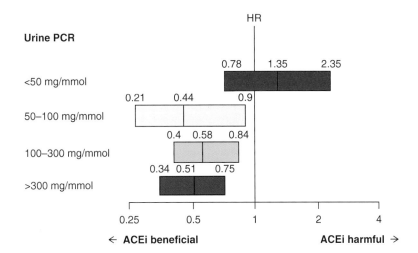

Fig. 3.1 ACEi and baseline urine PCR in non-diabetic proteinuria (Jafar et al. *Ann Int Med.* 2001;135:73–87)

of microalbuminuria is important for two reasons. Microalbuminuria is the earliest sign of diabetic nephropathy in patients with diabetes. Microalbuminuria may also occur in non-diabetic patients with vascular disease, possibly reflecting endothelial damage.

Q9 Why are microalbuminuria and proteinuria important when assessing patients with CKD?

Large population studies, studies of patients at risk of CKD e.g. people with diabetes and studies of patients with established CKD have all shown that microalbuminuria and proteinuria are independent risk factors not only for vascular disease but also for progressive renal failure. The risk of vascular disease is greater than the risk of progressive renal failure and the greater the level of proteinuria the higher is that risk. We note the latest NICE CKD guideline has lowered the threshold for clinically important proteinuria from an ACR >30 mg/mmol to an ACR >3 mg/mmol. It is too early to say how widely this new advice will be adopted.

Q10 What can be done to reduce risk in patients with microalbuminuria and proteinuria?

There are two key recommendations. The first is to control blood pressure and the second is to use an ACE inhibitor or angiotensin

receptor blocker as these drugs have both anti-hypertensive and anti-proteinuric properties. The NICE guideline on chronic kidney disease suggests that in people with CKD one should aim to keep the systolic pressure somewhere between 120 and 139 mmHg and a diastolic pressure less than 90 mmHg. A lower target of systolic pressure of between 120 and 129 mmHg with diastolic pressure less than 80 mmHg is recommended for people with CKD and diabetes, also in those with urine PCR >100 mg/mmol, We recognise that while such tight BP control might be desirable it is not usually achievable. NICE recommend that ACE inhibitors or angiotensin receptor blockers should now be considered as first line drug therapy for people with diabetes whose urine ACR exceeds 3 mg/mmol, for hypertensives with urine PCR >50 mg/mmol and for anyone with urine PCR >100 mg/mmol irrespective of their blood pressure. The figure above is a meta-analysis showing that ACE inhibitors have a beneficial effect on renal outcome in non-diabetics but only when urine PCR >50 mg/mmol (Fig. 3.1).

3.1 Objectives: Proteinuria

After reading this chapter you should be able to answer the following:

Q1 What is proteinuria and how is it classified?

Q2 How is proteinuria detected?

Q3 Discuss the advantages and limitations of the dipstick test for measuring urine protein.

Q4 What is Bence Jones proteinuria?

Q5 Why do we no longer recommend a 24 h urine collection for quantifying urine protein?

Q6 Discuss the advantages and limitations of a dipstick test for measuring urine protein.

Q7 ACR or PCR?

Q8 What do you understand by the term microalbuminuria?

Q9 Why are microalbuminuria and proteinuria important when assessing patients with CKD?

Q10 What can be done to reduce risk in patients with microalbuminuria and proteinuria?

Further Reading

1. Kidney Disease: Improving Global Outcomes (KDIGO) CKD Work Group. KDIGO 2012 clinical practice guideline for the evaluation and management of chronic kidney disease. Kidney Inter Suppl. 2013;3:1–150.
2. National Institute for Health and Care Excellence. Chronic kidney disease: early identification and management of chronic kidney disease in primary and secondary care. CG182. London: National Institute for Health and Care Excellence; 2014.

Q1 What is haematuria and how is it classified?

Haematuria simply means the presence of red blood cells in the urine. The Renal Association and the British Association of Urological Surgeons have recently recommended that haematuria is classified as visible (previously macroscopic) or non visible (previously microscopic). Non visible haematuria may be spurious, transient or persistent and also symptomatic (urgency, frequency, dysuria) or asymptomatic. Causes are usually urological but may also be renal – the figure shows a red cell cast in a patient with glomerular (renal) haematuria (Fig. 4.1).

Q2 What is meant by the term spurious haematuria?

The commonest cause of spurious haematuria is contamination of the urine specimen by menstrual blood loss. The term is also used to describe false positive dipstick tests which occur in rhabdomyolysis and haemoglobinuria because myoglobin and haemoglobin cross react with the chemical reagent on the test strip; and the red or pink urine that is sometimes seen with foods such as beetroot or drugs such as rifampicin.

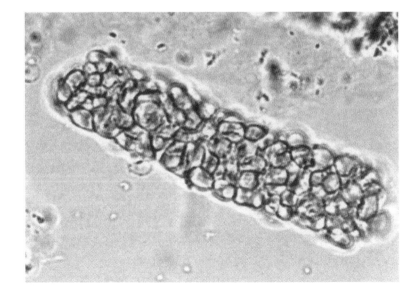

Fig. 4.1 Red cell cast. Urinary casts are cylindrical structures formed in the distal convoluted tubule & collecting ducts. Red cell casts are always pathological, and in cases of non-visible haematuria indicates glomerular damage

M. Findlay, C. Isles, *Clinical Companion in Nephrology*,
DOI 10.1007/978-3-319-14868-7_4, © Springer International Publishing Switzerland 2015

Q3 What are the causes of transient haematuria?

The two most important ones are urinary tract infection and vigorous exercise. Patients with suspected uncomplicated urinary infection should receive an appropriate empirical course of antibiotic e.g. trimethroprim followed by repeat urine dipstick 2 weeks later. If the follow up dipstick is negative no further tests are required. See below for what to do if the dipstick is positive

Q4 What is the risk of urological malignancy?

The likelihood of finding a urological malignancy in a patient with haematuria depends on age, gender and whether the haematuria is visible or non visible, as shown in the box below.

Box 4.1 Likelihood of Finding Malignancy Following a Presentation with Haematuria

	Non-visible (%)	Visible (%)
Male >40 year	8	24
Male <40 year	1	7
Female >40 year	4	19
Female <40 year	0	0

Khadra, et al. Analysis of 1930 patients with haematuria. *J Urol.* 2000;163:524–27; with permission from Elsevier

Q5 How should visible haematuria be investigated?

All adults with a single episode of visible haematuria should be referred to a urologist for renal imaging, usually ultrasound, and cystoscopy. A possible exception to the 'urology first' rule is the young adult <40 years of age who presents with recurrent haematuria lasting up to 48 h after an upper respiratory tract infection, in whom a diagnosis of IgA nephropathy is more likely.

Q6 What is the best way to confirm non visible haematuria?

Once spurious and transient causes of haematuria have been excluded then a reliable diagnosis of non-visible haematuria should be made by the urine dipstick test on a fresh specimen of urine. Trace positive haematuria can safely be regarded as negative as it represents less than three red blood cells per high power field on microscopy. Non visible haematuria in an asymptomatic patient is regarded as persistent if present in at least two of three dipstick tests over a period of 2 weeks. The NICE CKD guideline states that it is not necessary to confirm a positive dipstick test by urine microscopy if spurious causes can be excluded. The top test strip below is strongly positive for blood (fourth square from left) and also shows proteinuria (sixth from left) (Fig. 4.2).

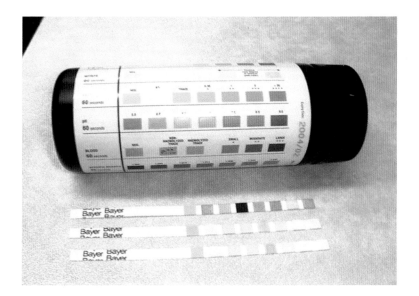

Fig. 4.2 Dipstick testing for haematuria

Q7 Having established that a patient has persistent non visible haematuria, what causes should you then consider?

These can also be classified as urological and renal. Again it is important not to miss a urological malignancy (as above) or an important renal disease (less common). IgA nephropathy is probably the most common of the renal causes. Other clues to an underlying renal cause are low or falling estimated GFR and/or urine PCR >50 mg/mmol. The urological and renal causes of non-visible haematuria are shown below.

Box 4.2 Causes of Non-visible Haematuria

Urological	Nephrological
Cancers of kidney, bladder or prostate	IgA nephropathy
Stones	Thin membrane disease
Urinary infections	Alport's syndrome
Benign tumours e.g. bladder papilloma	Other glomerular disease (usually with proteinuria)
Trauma	Inherited cystic disease e.g. polycystic kidney, medullary sponge kidney

Q8 What further investigations are indicated for a patient with persistent non visible haematuria?

This will depend on the age of the patient, the presence or absence of lower urinary tract symptoms (urgency, frequency, dysuria) and whether or not a renal cause is more likely than a urological one (renal impairment and proteinuria with urine PCR >50 mg/mmol). With these points in mind, the following three scenarios can be envisaged:

Box 4.3 Scenarios of Follow Up for Non Visible Haematuria

1. **Urology referral** – all patients with symptomatic non visible haematuria at any age and all patients with asymptomatic non visible haematuria aged ≥40 year. Assessment will usually be by ultrasound and cystoscopy.
2. **Nephrology referral** – consider for patients who have had a urological cause excluded, or have not met the referral criteria for a urological assessment. The need for a nephrology referral depends on factors other than simply the presence of haematuria and is recommended if there is renal impairment (eGFR <30 ml/min) or significant proteinuria (ACR ≥30 mg/mmol or PCR ≥50 mg/mmol)
3. **Follow up in primary care** – Younger patient (<40 years), asymptomatic and nothing else to suggest an underlying renal cause – follow up annually by blood pressure, urine dipstick, urea and electrolytes, urine ACR, referring to urology or nephrology as appropriate if the picture changes.

Q9 Should all patients with suspected IgA nephropathy be referred for renal biopsy?

Probably not. It makes sense to refer patients with visible haematuria who will probably want an explanation for something that they can see, and of course biopsy may be indicated if there is associated renal impairment and/or proteinuria. The risk of a biopsy probably outweighs the benefit of knowing the histology in patients with asymptomatic non-visible haematuria who have normal blood pressure, normal renal function and no proteinuria. In this situation it is common practice to apply the label "probable IgA nephropathy". Such patients do not necessarily need to attend specialist renal services, provided of course arrangements can be made for them to be followed annually in primary care.

4.1 Objectives: Haematuria

After reading this chapter you should be able to answer the following:

Q1 What is haematuria and how is it classified?

Q2 What is meant by the term spurious haematuria?

Q3 What are the causes of transient haematuria?

Q4 What is the risk of urological malignancy?

Q5 How should visible haematuria be investigated?

Q6 What is the best way to confirm non visible haematuria?

Q7 Having established that a patient has persistent non visible haematuria, what causes should you then consider?

Q8 What further investigations are indicated for a patient with persistent non visible haematuria?

Q9 Should all patients with suspected IgA nephropathy be referred for renal biopsy?

Further Reading

1. NICE CG182. Chronic kidney disease (partial update). Early identification and management of chronic kidney disease in adults in primary and secondary care, July 2014. http://www.nice.org.uk/guidance/cg182.
2. Renal Association and British Association of Urological Surgeons. Joint consensus statement on the initial assessment of haematuria, 2008. http://www.renal.org/docs/RA-BAUS_Haematuria_Consensus_Guidelines.pdf.

Part II

Disorders of Renal Metabolic Function

Hyponatraemia

Q1 Why do patients become hyponatraemic?

Hyponatraemia is a common electrolyte disturbance that is often difficult to diagnose and to manage. In all cases there is retention of water relative to sodium. It is usually mediated by ADH which is released appropriately (most cases) or inappropriately (SIADH).

Q2 Classify hyponatraemia by cause

Easily reversible causes include drugs, endocrine and psychogenic polydipsia. Thiazides are probably the commonest cause of hyponatraemia and are more likely than loop diuretics to cause hyponatraemia because they impair free water clearance to a greater extent. Other drug induced causes are carbamazepine, antidepressants and desmopressin. Endocrine causes include hypothyroidism, hypoadrenalism and hypopituitarism. Once these have been excluded it is conventional to classify patients by their extracellular fluid (ECF) volume status. Causes range from vomiting and diarrhoea (ECF reduced), nephrotic syndrome, cirrhosis and heart failure (ECF expanded) to the Syndrome of Inappropriate ADH secretion (SIADH) (euvolaemic).

Q3 Classify hyponatraemia by severity

Hyponatraemia may be mild, moderate or severe biochemically. Mild hyponatraemia is generally considered to mean serum sodium 130–135 mmol/L. Hyponatraemia is moderate with serum sodium 125–129 mmol/L and severe when serum sodium is less than 125 mmol/L.

Q4 How does hyponatraemia present clinically?

Most cases will be asymptomatic. The clinical features, when present, are those of cerebral oedema as water enters the brain. Initially there may be nausea, confusion and headache. Later there may be vomiting and cardiorespiratory distress leading ultimately to abnormal and deep somnolence, seizures and coma (GCS ≤8).

Q5 What is the relation between symptoms and duration of hyponatraemia?

Those at risk of cerebral oedema have acute hyponatraemia that develops within 48 h i.e. the brain swells because water moves across blood brain barrier before the brain has had time to adapt. Hyponatraemia is chronic if documented to exist for at least 48 h and considered to be chronic if the timing of onset is not known, unless there is clinical evidence of the contrary.

Q6 How should you investigate for the cause of hyponatraemia?

In many situations the cause of the hyponatraemia is evident from the history (e.g. recently commenced thiazide for hypertension) or the clinical examination (e.g. stigmata of chronic liver disease). In all cases the patient should have an accurate assessment of ECF volume status. The following five tests are will guide you to the aetiology of hyponatraemia, though all may not be necessary in every case (e.g. mild hyponatraemia following initiation of a thiazide):

M. Findlay, C. Isles, *Clinical Companion in Nephrology*,
DOI 10.1007/978-3-319-14868-7_5, © Springer International Publishing Switzerland 2015

1. Serum osmolality
2. Urine sodium
3. Urine osmolality
4. TFTs
5. Short synacthen test

Q7   Why is it important to check serum osmolality?

A measured serum osmolality <275 mOsm/kg always indicates hypotonic or true hyponatraemia. If serum osmolality is not low then artefactual, pseudo- and transient hyponatraemia should be considered. Artefactual hyponatraemia most commonly occurs when blood taken from the arm into which dextrose is being infused. Pseudohyponatraemia may occur in hyperlipidaemia and hyperproteinaemia (myeloma) because the amount of water in the plasma specimen is reduced by the volume occupied by the lipid or protein molecules. Transient hyponatraemia can also occur with acute hyperglycaemia which triggers a fall in serum sodium to maintain normal osmolality.

Q8   How does urine sodium help in diagnosis?

A low urine sodium ≤30 mmol/l suggests a low effective arterial blood volume and that the kidneys are doing their best to retain sodium in response to this. This is most frequently seen in hyponatraemic patients who are volume deplete but also in those with expanded ECF volume in whom effective arterial blood volume is also often low. Urine sodium >30 mmol/l is characteristic of SIADH because the patient is euvolaemic and has no reason to retain sodium. You should note however urine sodium may not be helpful in patients taking diuretics and in those with renal disease, in which circumstances you should consider all possible diagnoses as cause of hyponatraemia

Q9   How does urine osmolality help in diagnosis?

Urine osmolality is generally less useful than urine sodium in making a diagnosis. Urine osm <100 mosm/kg suggests psychogenic water drinking is the cause of hyponatraemia i.e. drinking too much water and passing large volumes dilute urine. Urine osm >700 mosm/kg means

that you are unlikely to correct hyponatraemia simply by water restriction.

Q10 How do you diagnose SIADH?

The criteria required to establish a diagnosis of SIADH are as shown in Box 5.1

Box 5.1 Criteria for SIADH
- Euvolaemia
- Low serum sodium <130 mmol/l
- Low serum osmolality <275 mosm/kg
- Urine osm >100 mosm/kg
- Urine Na typically >30 mmol/l
- No recent diuretic use
- Normal serum potassium, urea and urate
- Normal adrenal and thyroid function

Q11 Show a diagnostic approach to hyponatraemia that incorporates easily reversible causes, serum osmolality, urine sodium and assessment of ECF volume in a flow diagram

The flow diagram that follows shows the steps required to determine the cause of hyponatraemia (Fig. 5.1):

Q12 How do you treat hyponatraemia?

By considering and treating all reversible causes. In mild hyponatraemia (Na 130–135 mmol/l), there is no need to treat with the sole aim of increasing the serum sodium. Treatment of moderate and severe hyponatraemia will depend on a number of factors including cause, symptoms and whether the hyponatraemia is acute or chronic. Options include fluid restriction, saline 0.9 % and hypertonic saline 3.0 %. It is important not to correct severe hyponatraemia by more than 12 mmol/l in 24 h for fear of precipitating central pontine myelinolysis. We summarise a therapeutic approach to hyponatraemia in Appendix 1.

Q13 What is central pontine myelinolysis?

This is a neurological disorder that most frequently occurs if hyponatraemia is corrected too quickly. A rapid rise in serum sodium increases

Fig. 5.1 Diagnostic approach to hyponatraemia

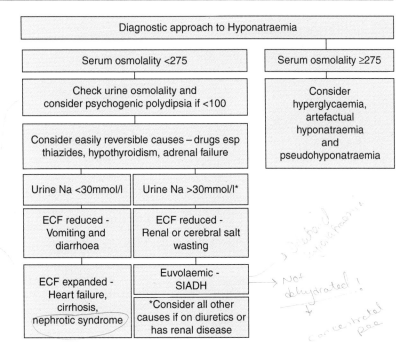

serum osmolality and leads to water moving out of the brain. This damages the protective myelin sheaths of certain neurons particularly those in the pons. The first symptoms of myelinolysis begin to appear 2–3 days after hyponatraemia is corrected, and include a reduced level of awareness, dysarthria and dysphagia. This may be followed by limb weakness, stiffness, impaired sensation, and difficulty with coordination. At its most severe, myelinolysis can lead to complete paralysis of all of the voluntary muscles in the body except for those that control the eyes (locked in syndrome), and death.

5.1   Objectives: Hyponatraemia

After reading this chapter you should be able to answer the following:

Q1   Why do patients become hyponatraemic?

Q2   Classify hyponatraemia by cause

Q3   Classify hyponatraemia by severity

Q4   How does hyponatraemia present clinically?

Q5   What is the relation between symptoms and duration of hyponatraemia?

Q6   How should you investigate for the cause of hyponatraemia?

Q7   Why is it important to check serum osmolality?

Q8   How does urine sodium help in diagnosis?

Q9   How does urine osmolality help in diagnosis?

Q10 How do you diagnose SIADH?

Q11 Show a diagnostic approach to hyponatraemia that incorporates easily reversible causes, serum osmolality, urine sodium and assessment of ECF volume in a flow diagram

Q12 How do you treat hyponatraemia?

Q13 What is central pontine myelinolysis?

Q1 How is serum potassium regulated?

We have described this already in Chap. 1. Briefly, serum potassium is kept in the range 3.5–5.4 mmol/l by a number of important mechanisms. Normal dietary K intake is 50–100 mmol per day. Ninety percent of body's 3,500 mmol K is intracellular and <1 % intravascular. Na/K pumps on cell membranes pump K into cells in exchange for Na under influence of insulin, beta agonists, alkalosis and aldosterone. Ninety percent excretion of K occurs through kidneys and only 10 % through colon unless patient has diarrhoea. Nearly all filtered K is reabsorbed and nearly all urine K is secreted by cells in the cortical collecting duct: aldosterone and alkalosis both lead to loss of K by these cells

Q2 Give the common causes of hypokalaemia

Common things occur commonly. Diuretics, nutritional causes including refeeding syndrome, vomiting, diarrhoea and acute illness were the five most common causes of hypokalaemia in a consecutive series of 61 patients with serum K <2.5 mmol/l seen in south west Scotland in 2010 (Fig. 6.1)

Artefact accounted for two of the patients in this series: one who had blood taken from a drip arm and another during a massive blood transfusion. One patient had renal tubular acidosis and

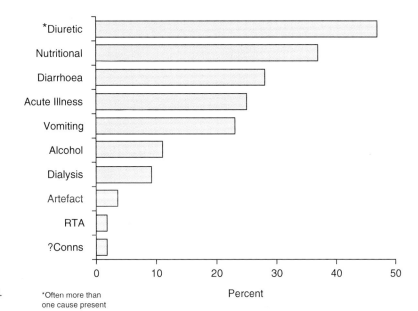

Fig. 6.1 Common causes of hypokalaemia (Reid, et al. Hypokalaemia: common things occur commonly – a retrospective survey. *J Roy Soc Med.* 2010;3:80–7)

*Often more than one cause present

one patient with hypertension and hypokalaemia probably had primary hyperaldosteronism but declined further investigations. There were no cases of Bartter's syndrome, Gitelman's syndrome, Liddle's syndrome or hypokalaemic periodic paralysis in this study.

Q3 What are the consequences of hypokalaemia?

The most serious effects are on the heart especially VT and potentiation of digoxin toxicity. Mild hypokalaemia in the range 3.0–3.5 mmol/l may well be asymptomatic. The more severe the hypokalaemia the more likely a patient will experience neuromuscular (weakness, myalgia, cramps, paralysis), gastrointestinal (constipation, ileus) and renal (polyuria) symptoms

Q4 How do you establish the cause of hypokalaemia?

If the cause is obvious e.g. diuretic, vomiting, diarrhoea then no further tests are required. In the absence of an obvious cause then the following simple tests will usually give the answer (Box 6.1)

Box 6.1 Investigation of Hypokalaemia
- Serum bicarbonate – most cases will be alkalotic. Hypokalaemia with acidosis raises possibility of renal tubular acidosis
- Serum PO_4 – often low in refeeding syndrome
- Serum magnesium – often low in hypokalaemia, esp when due to alcohol. Hypokalaemia may not correct until hypomagnesaemia corrected. Check magnesium if serum K <3.0 mmol/l
- Urine Potassium Creatinine Ratio – a high ratio suggests renal potassium wasting (see next question)

Q5 Is it ever worth measuring urine potassium?

Urine potassium can help you decide whether the cause of the hypokalaemia is renal or extrarenal when the cause is not obvious. You should bear in mind that vomiting causes hypokalaemia by renal potassium loss as vomit contains hydrochloric acid and very little potassium. The resulting alkalosis causes potassium to move into cells and leads to renal potassium loss at the level of the intercalated cell in the cortical collecting duct which retains hydrogen in exchange for potassium. The best way to check urine potassium is to send a urine sample to biochemistry for potassium:creatinine ratio. A ratio >1.5 suggests renal K wasting. It is obviously best to do this before starting potassium replacement therapy.

Q6 What if the cause of the hypokalaemia remains unclear?

There are a number of uncommon causes which might then need to be considered. Renal losses with normal BP raise the possibility of Bartter's and Gitelman's syndromes (patient will be alkalotic), or renal tubular acidosis (patient will be acidotic). Renal losses with hypertension point to Conn's syndrome (low plasma renin with high serum aldosterone), renovascular disease (renin and aldosterone both high), or Liddle's syndrome (renin and aldosterone both low). Textbooks devote a considerable amount of space to discussions of Bartter's, Gitelman's and Liddle's syndromes though they really are very rare (see Chap. 36).

Q7 How should you treat hypokalaemia?

Potassium replacement may be by oral supplements, potassium sparing diuretics or intravenously. The preparation given, the dose and the route of administration will be determined by the severity of the hypokalaemia and the presence or absence of symptoms (see Appendix 2)

6.1   Objectives: Hypokalaemia

After reading this chapter you should be able to answer the following:

Q1   How is serum potassium regulated?

Q2   Give the common causes of hypokalaemia

Q3   What are the consequences of hypokalaemia?

Q4   How do you establish the cause of hypokalaemia?

Q5   Is it ever worth measuring urine potassium?

Q6   What if the cause of the hypokalaemia remains unclear?

Q7   How should you treat hypokalaemia?

Hypocalcaemia and Hypercalcaemia

Q1 Where is calcium found in the body, what is the usual daily intake and normal serum level?

Ninety nine percent of the body's calcium is stored in bones. Less than 1 % circulates in the bloodstream. Usual calcium intake is 25 mmol or 1,000 mg/day, mainly in dairy products. Normal corrected total serum calcium in adults is 2.12–2.62 mmol/l. A correction factor is applied because serum calcium is part protein bound and part ionised. In practice this means the laboratory will add 0.02 mmol/l to the measured calcium level for every 1 g/l serum albumin is below 40 g/l.

Q2 How is serum calcium regulated?

Serum calcium is regulated by PTH, calcitonin and Vit D. PTH releases calcium from bone, calcitonin does the opposite while 1,25OHD increases absorption of calcium from the gut. Acidosis shifts the equilibrium between protein bound and ionised calcium towards ionised calcium while alkalosis has the opposite effect. This is the reason why both respiratory and metabolic alkalosis may cause symptoms of hypocalcaemia in the presence of a normal total serum calcium.

Q3 Give the causes of hypocalcaemia

There is no easy way to classify these. The commonest causes are hypoparathyroidism following parathyroidectomy or damage to parathyroid during total thyroidectomy, vitamin D deficiency, acute and chronic kidney disease. Very low calcium and magnesium may be seen in PPI associated hypocalcaemic hypomagnesaemic hypoparathyroidism. These and other less common causes are summarized in Box 7.1

Box 7.1 Causes of Hypocalcaemia
- Low PTH – following thyroid or parathyroid surgery
- High PTH (secondary hyperparathyroidism in response to hypocalcaemia) – vitamin D deficiency, acute and chronic kidney disease
- Drugs – biphosphonates, cinacalcet, PPIs (hypocalcaemic hypomagnesaemic hypoparathyroidism)
- Miscellaneous e.g. alkalosis, cytotoxic drugs, pancreatitis, rhabdomyolysis, large volume blood transfusion

---

Q4 How may hypocalcaemia present clinically?

Symptoms typically develop when adjusted calcium falls below 1.9 mmol/l but patients may be asymptomatic if rate of fall is slow. Clinical evidence of hypocalcaemia includes perioral and digital paraesthesia, muscle spasm (tetany) including carpopedal spasm and laryngospasm. Trousseau's sign – inflation of sphygmomanometer cuff above systolic pressure for 3 min induces

M. Findlay, C. Isles, *Clinical Companion in Nephrology*,
DOI 10.1007/978-3-319-14868-7_7, © Springer International Publishing Switzerland 2015

tetanic spasm of fingers and wrist, and Chvostek's sign – gentle tapping over the facial nerve induces twitching of the facial muscles – may both be positive. Prolonged QT interval may lead to ventricular arrhythmias. Seizures may occur if hypocalcaemia is severe or during over rapid correction of acidosis (because this lowers serum ionised calcium).

Q5 What investigations should be undertaken for hypocalcaemia?

Acute hypocalcaemia can be life threatening and because of this investigations can be organised and treatment started if necessary before the results are back. Baseline tests should include U&E with serum phosphate, magnesium, PTH and 25 hydroxy vitamin D. An ECG should be performed for prolonged QT interval and ventricular dysrhythmias.

Q6 When and how should hypocalcaemia be treated?

This depends on the severity of hypocalcaemia and whether or not symptoms are present. Options are Sandocal 1000 orally (each tab contains 25 mmol elemental calcium) or calcium gluconate 10 % IV (10 ml vial contains 2.3 mmol elemental calcium). Alfacalcidol, the active form of vitamin D, is likely to be required for surgical hypocalcaemia and for the hypocalcaemia of renal failure. For details see Appendix 3.

Q7 Give the causes of hypercalcaemia

Ninety percent of causes are due to malignancy or primary hyperparathyroidism. Malignancies that commonly cause hypercalcaemia are breast (parathyroid related protein), lung (ectopic PTH) and myeloma (release of osteoclastic activating factors). All other causes are much less common. They include drugs e.g. vitamin D (increased absorption calcium from gut), lithium (increased secretion PTH) and thiazides (reduced tubular excretion calcium), sarcoidosis (hydroxylation of vitamin D in granulomas), thyrotoxicosis (increased osteoclastic activity), milk alkali syndrome and tertiary hyperparathyroidism

Box 7.2 Causes of Hypercalcaemia
- Malignancy (including myeloma)
- Primary hyperparathyroidism
- Drugs – e.g. vitamin D, lithium, thiazides
- Sarcoidosis
- Thyrotoxicosis
- Milk/alkali syndrome
- Tertiary hyperparathryoidism

Q8 How may hypercalcaemia present clinically?

Clinical presentation may be remembered by the mnemonic 'bones, stones, abdominal groans, psychic moans, thrones and hypertones'. Bones refers to bone related complications such as osteoporosis, stones to renal colic, abdominal groans to peptic ulcer, psychic moans to depression, thrones to polyuria and constipation and hypertones to hypertension. In reality 50 % patients are asymptomatic and many have non-specific symptoms e.g. lethargy and malaise. Acute severe hypercalcaemia is a medical emergency and may present with shock, coma and renal failure.

Q9 How should you investigate hypercalcaemia?

The most useful investigation is plasma PTH. If PTH is detectable or increased then primary hyperparathyroidism is the probable diagnosis. If PTH is decreased or undetectable and no other cause is apparent then malignancy with or without bony metastases is likely. Unless the source of tumour is obvious then screen for malignancy with CXR, myeloma screen and CT chest abdo pelvis as appropriate.

Q10 When and how should hypercalcaemia be treated?

This depends on the severity of hypercalcaemia and whether or not symptoms are present. The first priority is to rehydrate with intravenous saline which has the added benefit of promoting calciuresis. IV biphophonates are then indicated to inhibit bone resorption and are particularly effective in the hypercalcaemia of malignancy. For details see Appendix 4.

7.1   Objectives: Hypocalcaemia and Hypercalcaemia

After reading this chapter you should be able to answer the following:

Q1   Where is calcium found in the body, what is the usual daily intake and normal serum level?

Q2   How is serum calcium regulated?

Q3   Give the causes of hypocalcaemia

Q4   How may hypocalcaemia present clinically?

Q5   What investigations should be undertaken for hypocalcaemia?

Q6   When and how should hypocalcaemia be treated?

Q7   Give the causes of hypercalcaemia

Q8   How may hypercalcaemia present clinically?

Q9   How should you investigate hypercalcaemia?

Q10   When and how should hypercalcaemia be treated?

Hypophosphataemia and Hypomagnesaemia

8

Q1 Where is phosphate found in the body, what is the usual daily intake and normal serum level?

About 85 % of body's phosphorus is found in bone. The rest is stored intracellularly in tissues. It is therefore difficult to assess body stores from serum levels. Usual dietary phosphate intake is 30–50 mmol/day, mainly in dairy products. The reference range for serum phosphate in adults is 0.7–1.4 mmol/l.

Q2 Give the causes of hypophosphataemia

These can be considered under three headings, summarised in the box below.

> **Box 8.1 Causes of Hypophosphatemia**
> - Inadequate intake e.g. poor diet from alcoholism, inadequate replacement during prolonged parenteral nutrition
> - Increased renal losses e.g. primary hyperparathyroidism, vitamin D deficiency, hypomagnesaemia
> - Transcellular shift e.g. refeeding syndrome, treatment of DKA, severe respiratory alkalosis,

Q3 How may hypophosphataemia present clinically?

Most patients with hypophosphataemia have no specific symptoms. When symptoms do occur then muscle weakness, bone pain, rhabdomyolysis, confusion and hallucinations are the most common presenting features. Serum $PO_4 < 0.3$ mmol/l is a medical emergency with risk of seizures, focal neurological deficits and heart failure, respiratory failure (due to weakness of the diaphragm), a proximal myopathy, dysphagia and ileus in addition to above.

Q4 When and how should hypophosphataemia be treated?

This depends on the severity of hypophosphataemia and whether or not symptoms are present. Options are Phosphate-Sandoz orally (each tab contains 16 mmol phosphate) or Addiphos IV (20 ml vial contains 40 mmol phosphate). For details see Appendix 5.

Q5 Where is magnesium found in the body, what is the usual daily intake and normal serum level?

The body contains around 1,000 mmol Mg, 50–60 % of which is in bone and the rest in soft tissues which means that serum levels do not necessarily reflect body stores. Mg is a cofactor in more than 300 enzyme systems that regulate, among other things, muscle and nerve function. Usual magnesium intake is 15–20 mmol per day. Normal serum level is 0.7–1.0 mmol/l.

Q6 Give the causes of hypomagnesaemia?

The three main mechanisms that lead to hypomagnesaemia are inadequate intake, gastrointestinal and renal losses. These are summarised in the following box.

M. Findlay, C. Isles, *Clinical Companion in Nephrology*, DOI 10.1007/978-3-319-14868-7_8, © Springer International Publishing Switzerland 2015

Box 8.2 Causes of Hypomagnesaemia
- Inadequate intake e.g. poor diet from alcoholism
- Gastrointestinal losses e.g. malabsorption, chronic diarrhea and pancreatitis
- Renal losses – aminoglycosides, platinum, cyclosporine and high dose combination diuretic therapy
- Other e.g. PPIs may cause hypocalcaemic hypomagnesaemic hypoparathyroidism

Q7 How may hypomagnesaemia present clinically?

Clinical features are neuromuscular and cardiovascular. Neuromuscular symptoms are paraesthesia, muscle cramps, irritability and confusion, while cardiovascular effects include atrial and ventricular dysrhythmias. Mg deficiency is often associated with other electrolyte deficiencies especially hypocalcaemia, hypokalaemia and hypophosphataemia, hence the need to check serum Mg if serum Ca, K or PO_4 are low

Q8 When and how should hypomagnesaemia be treated?

Again this depends on the severity of the electrolyte upset and whether or not symptoms are present. Options are magnesium glycerophosphate orally (each tab contains 4 mmol magnesium) or magnesium sulphate IV (10 ml of 50 % solution contains 20 mmol magnesium). For details see Appendix 5.

8.1 Objectives: Hypophosphataemia and Hypomagnesaemia

After reading this chapter you should be able to answer the following:

Q1 Where is phosphate found in the body, what is the usual daily intake and normal serum level?

Q2 Give the causes of hypophosphataemia

Q3 How may hypophosphataemia present clinically?

Q4 When and how should hypophosphataemia be treated?

Q5 Where is magnesium found in the body, what is the usual daily intake and normal serum level?

Q6 Give the causes of hypomagnesaemia?

Q7 How may hypomagnesaemia present clinically?

Q8 When and how should hypomagnesaemia be treated?

Q1 How do you diagnose an acid-base disorder?

You will be able to diagnose acid-base disorders correctly by measuring hydrogen ion concentration (normal range 35–45 nmol/l) or pH (normal range 7.36–7.44), $PaCO_2$ (normal range 4.6–6.0 kPa) and serum bicarbonate (normal range 22–27 mmol/l) on an arterial blood gas sample, which will also give you PaO_2 and lactate. Venous gases can be used in an emergency if an arterial sample is not possible and will give reliable measurements of H^+, $PaCO_2$ and bicarbonate provided you use a blood gas tube.

Q2 There are only four disorders of acid-base balance. What are they?

These are metabolic acidosis, metabolic alkalosis, respiratory acidosis and respiratory alkalosis. Patients are considered to be acidotic if their H^+ concentration >45 kPa or pH <7.36 and alkalotic when H+ <35 kPa or pH >7.44. If the patient is acidotic and the $PaCO_2$ is increased this is a

respiratory acidosis whereas if $PaCO_2$ is normal this is a metabolic acidosis. If the patient is alkalotic and the $PaCO_2$ is reduced this is a respiratory alkalosis whereas if $PaCO_2$ is normal this is a metabolic alkalosis. We summarise these disturbances and the compensatory changes that follow in Table 9.1. Compensatory changes are either pulmonary (affecting ventilation) or renal (affecting bicarbonate reabsorption). Their purpose is to return H+ concentration towards normal so far as is possible.

Q3 How do you diagnose metabolic acidosis?

If the patient is acidotic and the $PaCO_2$ is normal this is a metabolic acidosis. Patients compensate for this by blowing off CO_2 which often leads to deep respirations e.g. the Kussmaul breathing of DKA. Further assessment requires that you calculate the anion gap which enables you to determine whether the patient has normal or high anion gap metabolic acidosis.

Table 9.1 The four disorders of acid-base balance

H+	Interpretation	CO_2	Acid-base disorder	Compensatory change
Increased	Acidotic	Normal or low	Metabolic acidosis	Respiratory: Fall in CO_2
		High	Respiratory acidosis	Metabolic: Rise in bicarb
Decreased	Alkalotic	Normal or high	Metabolic alkalosis	Respiratory: Rise in CO_2
		Low	Respiratory alkalosis	Metabolic: Fall in bicarb

M. Findlay, C. Isles, *Clinical Companion in Nephrology*,
DOI 10.1007/978-3-319-14868-7_9, © Springer International Publishing Switzerland 2015

Q4   What is meant by the term anion gap?

The anion gap is the difference between measured cations (positively charged) and measured anions (negatively charged). What this means is that you subtract serum bicarbonate and chloride from serum sodium and potassium, as shown:

$$\text{normal anion gap} = (\text{serum Na} + \text{K}) - (\text{serum bicarbonate} + \text{chloride}) = 6 - 16\,\text{mmol}/\text{l}$$

Q5   What are the causes of a high anion gap acidosis?

The anion gap is high when the cause of the acidosis is excess acid production as in D**KA**, **U**raemia, **S**alicylate overdose, **S**epsis, **M**ethanol or ethylene glycol poisoning, **A**lcoholic ketoacidosis, **L**actic acidosis. Lactic acidosis is commonly due to sepsis and shock. The diagnosis is likely if blood lactate >2 on a blood gas sample. This and the other causes of a high anion gap acidosis are readily remembered using the **KUSSMAL** mnemonic.

Q6   What are the causes of a normal anion gap acidosis?

The anion gap is normal when the cause is loss of bicarbonate. In most cases this leads to a hyperchloraemic acidosis as chloride is retained in order to maintain electroneutrality. Bicarbonate loss can be from the gut or the kidney. The commonest cause is diarrhoea. Other causes of gut bicarbonate loss are villous adenoma and small intestine, pancreatic or biliary drains or fistulae. The renal causes are renal tubular acidosis, acetazolamide and urinary diversion procedures, especially ureterosigmoidostomy.

Q7   Saline 0.9 % may also cause a hyperchloraemic acidosis. Why ?

Infusion of large volumes of saline 0.9 % is another important cause of hyperchloraemic acidosis. This is most easily thought of as occurring because of the large chloride load and the rapid dilution of serum bicarbonate by saline. It is one of the reasons why Hartmann's is the crystalloid of choice when prescribing replacement fluid (see Chap. 17).

Q8   What do you need to know about renal tubular acidosis?

The renal tubular acidoses are a heterogeneous group of disorders characterised by normal anion gap hyperchloraemic acidosis. Type 1 RTA (distal RTA) is characterised by failure of hydrogen ion secretion by the distal tubule while type 2 RTA (proximal RTA) occurs when the proximal tubules are unable to reabsorb bicarbonate. Both are associated with hypokalaemia. Type 3 RTA is a vanishingly rare combination of types 1 and 2 RTA while type 4 RTA is usually due to aldosterone deficiency and is associated with hyperkalaemia. Type 4 RTA is the commonest RTA and is worth being aware of.

Q9   How would you recognise type 4 RTA and what should you do about it?

The clue to the presence of type 4 RTA is more hyperkalaemia and acidosis than you would expect for the serum creatinine concentration e.g. serum K is around 6 mmol/l and serum bicarbonate 18 mmol/l when serum creatinine is only 170 umol/l. This syndrome, which is commonly seen in people with diabetes, is sometimes known as hyporeninaemic hypoaldosteronism reflecting the fact that the underlying problem may be failure of the renin response to sodium depletion. Hypoaldosteronism means that less potassium and hydrogen are secreted into the tubules. Treatment with a loop diuretic is usually effective.

Q10   How would you recognise metabolic alkalosis, what are its causes and what should you do about it?

If the patient is alkalotic and $PaCO_2$ is normal then this is a metabolic alkalosis. The compensatory mechanism is hypoventilation which in severe cases can lead to significant CO_2 retention and hypoxaemia. Common causes include vomiting due to gastric outlet obstruction and diuretic therapy causing hypokalaemia both of which are associated with raised serum bicarbonate. Serum chloride is low in gastric outlet obstruction which is a major clue to this disorder. Treatment is that of the underlying cause with correction of hypokalaemia as required (see Chap. 6).

Q11   How would you recognise respiratory acidosis, what are its causes and what should you do about it?

If the patient is acidotic and the $PaCO_2$ is increased then this is a respiratory acidosis. The commonest cause is COPD with ventilatory failure but any cause of ventilatory failure will produce this picture e.g. respiratory depression due to opiates/sedatives or neuromuscular disorders. Serum bicarbonate is normal in acute respiratory acidosis and rises as a compensatory mechanism in chronic respiratory acidosis. Treatment is by improving ventilation e.g. by non-invasive ventilation (NIV) in exacerbations of COPD.

Q12   How would you recognise respiratory alkalosis, what are its causes and what should you do about it?

If the patient is alkalotic and the $PaCO_2$ is reduced then this is a respiratory alkalosis. The kidney compensates by reducing bicarbonate reabsorption so that serum bicarbonate falls. Any cause of hyperventilation may cause a respiratory alkalosis e.g. anxiety, LVF, pneumonia and pulmonary embolism. Hyperventilation due to panic attacks causes a transient respiratory alkalosis which is dominated by the symptoms of acute hypocalcaemia. This is because the alkalosis shifts the equilibrium between ionised and non-ionised calcium in favour of non-ionised calcium, leading to tingling in both hands and numbness around the mouth. Once again, treatment of respiratory alkalosis is that of the underlying condition.

9.1   Objectives: Acid-Base Balance

After reading this chapter you should be able to answer the following:

Q1   How do you diagnose an acid-base disorder?

Q2   There are only four disorders of acid-base balance. What are they?

Q3   How do you diagnose metabolic acidosis?

Q4   What is meant by the term anion gap?

Q5   What are the causes of a high anion gap acidosis?

Q6   What are the causes of a normal anion gap acidosis?

Q7   Saline 0.9 % may also cause a hyperchloraemic acidosis. Why ?

Q8   What do you need to know about renal tubular acidosis

Q9   How would you recognise type 4 RTA and what should you do about it?

Q10   How would you recognise metabolic alkalosis, what are its causes and what should you do about it?

Q11   How would you recognise respiratory acidosis, what are its causes and what should you do about it?

Q12   How would you recognise respiratory alkalosis, what are its causes and what should you do about it?

Part III

Acute Kidney Injury

Q1 What is meant by the term acute kidney injury?

AKI describes conditions in which the kidney loses function over hours and days rather than months and years (this makes it distinct from chronic kidney disease). AKI is usually but not always associated with oliguria, defined as urine volume less than 0.5 ml/kg/h (approximately 30 ml/h). Consensus definitions proposed by the Acute Dialysis Quality Initiative (ADQI) and the Acute Kidney Injury Network (AKIN) have been merged to produce a new definition and staging system as shown in the box below:

The baseline creatinine is the lowest value within 3 months of the episode of AKI. If a baseline is not available, and AKI is suspected, then repeat the creatinine in 24 h. If there is no baseline within 3 months and the patient recovers then you can use the lowest creatinine during recovery to stage the severity of AKI retrospectively

Q2 Give a clinical approach to the diagnosis of unexplained renal failure.

There are numerous ways of doing this. The 'pre-renal, renal, post-renal' approach is a good place to start but still requires a way of remembering what are the pre-renal, renal and post-renal causes (Fig. 10.1).

Box 10.1 Definitions of AKI

Stage	Serum creatinine criteria	Urine output criteria
1	Increase ≥26 umol/l or increase 1.5–1.9× from baseline	<0.5 ml/kg/h for >6 consecutive hours
2	Increase 2–2.9× from baseline	>12 h
3	Increase ≥3× or increase ≥354 umol/l or RRT irrespective of stage	<0.3 ml/kg/h for >24 h or anuria for >12 h

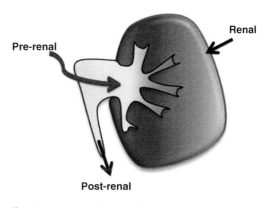

Fig. 10.1 Causes of acute kidney injury

M. Findlay, C. Isles, *Clinical Companion in Nephrology*,
DOI 10.1007/978-3-319-14868-7_10, © Springer International Publishing Switzerland 2015

The lists given in standard textbooks are usually long and are sometimes unhelpful in that they do not differentiate causes of acute kidney injury that are extremely common from those that are vanishingly rare. A practical way of approaching the diagnosis of acute kidney injury is to consider the following five questions:

Box 10.2 The Five Clinical Questions of AKI

Q1 Is it acute, acute on chronic or chronic presenting acutely?

Q2 Are there risk factors for acute tubular necrosis?

Q3 Is there evidence of obstruction?

Q4 Is there renal inflammation?

Q5 Are there any pointers to other causes of AKI?

Q3 How can you tell if AKI is acute or acute on chronic?

This question is usually answered by reviewing previous blood results. Most would agree that if a patient has had a serum creatinine greater than 150 μmol/l for over 3 months before presentation with AKI, then this is likely to be acute on chronic kidney disease. In the absence of previous blood results renal ultrasound can assess for chronicity. A renal ultrasound which shows bilateral small kidneys (each less than 9 cm in bipolar diameter) implies CKD.

Q4 What is meant by chronic presenting acutely?

Chronic Kidney Disease Presenting Acutely (CKDPA aka "Crash Landing") is important to recognise because these patients may require dialysis within a week of first presentation and have little time to prepare for the demanding treatment that lies ahead. We describe a case below:

Case Report

A 17-year-old girl presented to her general practitioner with 4 weeks of progressively worsening nausea and vomiting, superimposed on a few months of general malaise. Initially she vomited twice a day but by the end of the 4 weeks she was vomiting all the time. This was associated with epigastric pain, anorexia and weight loss of approximately 1 stone. Her symptoms did not respond to omeprazole and led to referral for endoscopy. While awaiting her endoscopy, her general practitioner noted that she looked pale and sent off bloods, which revealed haemoglobin, 46 g/l with serum potassium, 8.2 mmol/l, serum bicarbonate, 11 mmol/l, blood urea, 93.3 mmol/l and serum creatinine, 3,737 μmol/l. She had her first dialysis that evening. Renal biopsy showed that the cause of her renal failure was chronic interstitial nephritis. She remained dialysis dependent and subsequently received a live donor transplant from her mother.

Reproduced from Wolfe M, et al. Chronic kidney disease presenting acutely: presentation, clinical features and outcome of patients with irreversible chronic kidney disease who require dialysis immediately. *Postgrad Med J*. 2010;86:405–8, with permission from BMJ Publishing Group Ltd

The clue to the diagnosis is the severity both of the anaemia and the uraemia. The only way the haemoglobin could have fallen this far or the urea to have risen that high without presenting earlier is for the chronic kidney disease to have evolved slowly over a period of months or years.

Q5 What do you understand by the term acute tubular necrosis (ATN)?

ATN is what happens if we fail to restore renal perfusion quickly enough in a patient with pre-renal ARF. A patient with ATN usually becomes dialysis dependent for a period of time until the tubules regenerate. This can take anything from 3 days to 3 months depending on the severity of the insult.

Q6 What are the four main risk factors for acute tubular necrosis?

Essentially these are the pre-renal causes of AKI which together account for the majority of cases of AKI. You can assess the four reversible factors by asking the following questions:

1. **Are they dry?**
2. **Are they wet?**
3. **Are they infected?**
4. **Are they taking a nephrotoxic drug?**

Patients with AKI commonly have more than one pre-renal cause for their kidney injury. Sepsis and nephrotoxic drugs are discussed in more detail here, with 'dry' (i.e. hypovolaemia of any cause) and 'wet' (i.e. cardiac failure and other pathologies associated with ECF overload) being covered in the chapters on fluid management and cardiorenal failure. We recognise that not all nephrotoxins cause pre-renal AKI (e.g. gentamicin) but it is convenient nevertheless to think of them as a group of reversible causes.

Q7 Give ten important nephrotoxins.

Medical students often start answering this question by naming gentamicin. This commonly causes AKI at high serum levels but is not an important cause of AKI in the population because its use is limited to a small group of extremely sick patients in hospital. The top ten frequently encountered nephrotoxic drugs are probably:

> **Box 10.3 Commonly Encountered Nephrotoxins**
> - ACE inhibitors
> - Angiotensin receptor blockers
> - NSAIDs
> - Radio-contrast agents
> - Calcineurin inhibitors
> - Aminoglycosides
> - Vancomycin
> - Lithium
> - Proton pump inhibitors (Interstitial Nephritis)
> - Overdose of Paracetamol

Q8 How do ACEI and ARBs cause AKI?

Angiotensin II constricts the efferent arteriole and is responsible for maintaining glomerular capillary pressure whenever renal perfusion is reduced (below, left). Giving an ACE inhibitor prevents the formation of angiotensin II leading to loss of efferent arteriolar constriction and a fall in GFR (below, right). If the fall in GFR is marked then AKI will occur. This is commonly seen in patients who develop vomiting and diarrhoea while taking an ACE inhibitor. Exactly the same problem can arise with angiotensin receptors blockers (ARBs) which block the action of angiotensin II (Fig. 10.2).

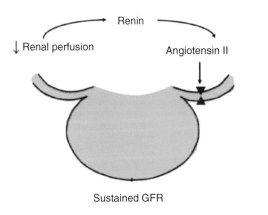 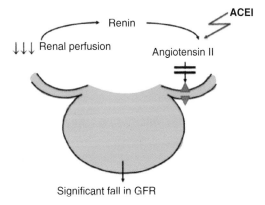

Fig. 10.2 Mechanism of AKI by ACE inhibitors in the presence of reduced renal perfusion

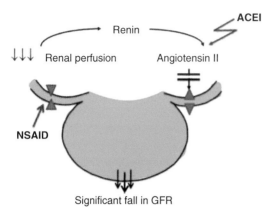

Significant fall in GFR

Fig. 10.3 Mechanism of ACEi and NSAID induced AKI

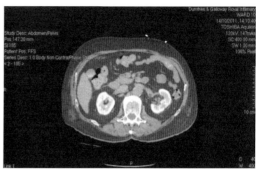

Fig. 10.4 CT image of kidneys following contrast with visible uptake in the renal cortex

Q9 How do NSAIDs cause AKI?

These drugs inhibit prostaglandins which are responsible for dilating the afferent arteriole. NSAIDs impair renal perfusion by constricting the afferent arteriole. The combination of an NSAID and an ACE inhibitor can be very bad news for the kidney and is sometimes referred to as a 'double whammy' (Fig. 10.3).

Q10 Who is most at risk of contrast nephropathy?

The contrast agents used in some x-rays – for example CT renal angiogram and coronary angiography are toxic to the renal tubules and can cause acute kidney injury. The risk is higher in the elderly, people with diabetes, patients taking diuretics, those who are dehydrated from any cause and patients with pre-existing renal failure. The abdominal CT scan shown below was taken 48 h after a coronary angiogram in a patient who had developed AKI. The bright white appearance to the kidneys demonstrates quite clearly that the contrast has been taken up by and persisted in the renal cortex (Fig. 10.4).

Q11 What steps might you take to prevent contrast nephropathy?

Prevention of Contrast Induced Nephropathy (CIN) is the most effective treatment although no universally accepted prevention strategy exists. If a contrast based CT scan is felt necessary, most agree that in those at risk (eGFR <60 ml/min) pre-hydration with 500–1,000 mL of crystalloid and cessation of potential nephrotoxins are advisable. Some studies have shown a slight reduction in the risk of CIN by giving N-acetylcysteine (NAC) orally. Other than a bitter taste this has no significant adverse effects. Therefore in the 'Higher risk' patients (i.e. those with an eGFR <30 or eGFR <45 with diabetes or myeloma) some nephrologists would recommend NAC 1,200 mg twice daily on the day before and the day of the procedure.

Q12 Explain why ciclosporin & tacrolimus – two drugs commonly used in transplantation – are double edged swords.

The calcineurin inhibitors, ciclosporin and tacrolimus, are required to prevent rejection in patients with renal transplants but both are nephrotoxic at high levels. For this reason monitoring of these drugs (trough serum levels) is carried out – adjusting the dose according to well defined target ranges. If a transplanted patient is found to have a sudden increase in their serum creatinine with a high trough level of either drug then a dose reduction will frequently improve their renal function.

Q13 What clinical features might suggest obstructive uropathy was the cause of AKI?

Obstructive uropathy should be suspected in anyone with a history of prostatic disease, bladder carcinoma, colon cancer or cervical cancer. Prostatic disease may be benign or malignant. Benign prostatic hypertrophy usually presents with nocturia, difficulty starting, poor stream and dribbling towards the end of micturition, and tends to cause bladder neck obstruction (bladder is full on ultrasound) while prostatic cancer more commonly invades the base of the bladder leading to obstruction at both ureters (bladder empty on ultrasound). Other important clues to obstructive uropathy are a history of renal stones. Bear in mind stone disease must be bilateral or present in a patient with a solitary kidney in order to cause AKI. Complete anuria suggests obstruction but its absence does not exclude, as patients with partial obstruction can have polyuria and those with near complete obstruction may have urinary retention with overflow. Retroperitoneal fibrosis is another important cause of obstructive uropathy though there are not usually any clinical clues to this diagnosis.

Q14 How might clinical examination suggest a diagnosis of obstructive uropathy?

The most useful clinical sign is a palpable bladder with increased bladder dullness which, if present, frequently means the bladder contains at least a litre of urine. A palpable bladder is easily detected in a slim patient but may not be so if the patient is obese. Agitation in an elderly male should always lead the hand to the lower abdomen, as elderly men with urinary retention frequently have no urinary symptoms to speak of, though they can certainly become agitated. AKI that either develops in or does not improve with a urinary catheter should alert the clinician to the possibility that the catheter is blocked or in the wrong position. A portable bladder scanner can

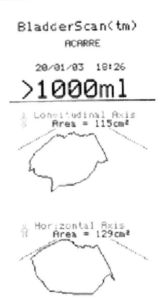

Fig. 10.5 Bladder scan of urinary retention

be a most useful diagnostic tool in these circumstances (Fig. 10.5)

Q15 How is the diagnosis of obstructive uropathy usually confirmed?

By renal ultrasound which will normally show pelvicalyceal dilatation, but will be falsely negative in around 5 % of cases. False negative results may be found in patients who are dehydrated and in those with a degree of underlying chronic kidney disease whose kidneys have started to fibrose and whose pelvi-calyceal systems cannot therefore dilate. The take home message therefore is that clinicians should consider obstruction as the likely cause of AKI even if the ultrasound shows no upper tract dilatation, in circumstances where obstruction is likely. Similarly, you should always consider the possibility that obstruction is the cause of AKI in a patient with a urinary catheter, particularly after a difficult catheterisation, even if the catheter appears to be draining normally as the patient may have retention with overflow (Fig. 10.6).

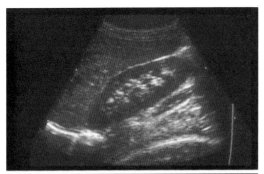

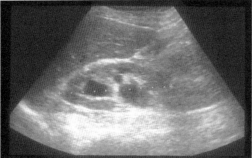

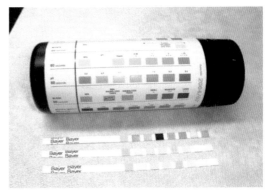

Fig. 10.7 Urine dipstick strongly positive for blood and protein (*top strip*)

renal vasculitis and interstitial nephritis is the presence of significant proteinuria and haematuria on dipstick testing. One plus protein and a small amount of haematuria is a fairly non-specific finding in AKI but heavy proteinuria and/or a strongly positive dipstick for haematuria should always raise the possibility of renal inflammation (Fig. 10.7).

Fig. 10.6 Two renal ultrasound images comparing images of a normal kidney (*top*) and a hydronephrotic kidney (*bottom*)

Q16 What are the causes of renal inflammation and what clues may there be that this is present?

The two important causes of renal inflammation are systemic vasculitis and interstitial nephritis. Rapidly progressive glomerulonephritis due to systemic vasculitis is covered elsewhere (Chap. 19). The clinical clue is 'renal failure plus' where the 'plus' usually means either lung involvement as in pulmonary renal syndrome or skin involvement with a vasculitic rash. Interstitial nephritis is generally either idiopathic or secondary to drugs such as antibiotics, non-steroidal anti-inflammatories and proton pump inhibitors. Drug induced acute interstitial nephritis is commonly but not always associated with a skin rash and eosinophilia. The diagnosis can only be made by renal biopsy. Treatment is by drug withdrawal followed by prednisolone 1 mg/kg (maximum 60 mg) daily for 1 month in the first instance. Steroids should be started promptly after diagnosis to avoid subsequent interstitial fibrosis and an incomplete recovery of renal function. An important and often overlooked clinical clue to both

Q17 What are the other important causes of AKI and describe how you might recognise these?

The specific causes of acute kidney injury are covered in more detail in the next chapter. If you prefer a pathophysiological approach you could describe the 'renal' causes as:

> **Box 10.4 Intrarenal Causes of Acute Kidney Injury**
> **Tubular** – acute tubular necrosis
> **Glomerular** – systemic vasculitis
> **Interstitial** – interstitial nephritis
> **Vascular** – renovascular, athero-embolism, thrombotic microangiopathy

An alternative approach, which we favour, is to consider the causes of AKI by the frequency with which they occur. In an analysis of 396 cases of AKI requiring dialysis and presenting to our district general hospital in the west of Scotland,

298 were AKI only while 98 (25 %) had acute on chronic kidney disease. 75 % of the AKI only cases were due to one or more of the pre-renal or post-renal causes already described. The remaining 25 % cases of AKI only were caused by a diverse group of conditions including pancreatitis, hepatorenal syndrome, atheroembolism, renovascular, rhabdomyolysis, myeloma, malignant hypertension, interstitial nephritis, infiltration by lymphoma, systemic vasculitis, thrombotic microangiopathy and tumour lysis syndrome, which were mostly 'renal' and for which the acronym PHARMACIST can be applied (note that this list also includes acute on chronic and CKD presenting acutely as already discussed).

	Cause	Clue
I	Interstitial nephritis	Suspect in any AKI especially if has taken antibiotic, NSAID, PPI
	Infiltrative	e.g. parenchymal infiltration by lymphoma
S	Systemic vasculitis[a]	Suspect if 'renal failure plus', especially pulmonary-renal, vasculitic skin rash.
T	Thrombotic microangiopathy	Triad of AKI with thrombocytopenia and haemolysis with red cell fragments
	Tumour lysis syndrome	AKI following chemotherapy with high urate, phosphate and potassium

[a]Each of these diagnoses are discussed in more detail in later chapters

Box 10.5 PHARMACIST Acronym for Intra-renal Causes of Acute Kidney Injury

	Cause	Clue
P	Pancreatitis	Severe upper abdominal pain with serum amylase >300 u/l
H	Hepato-renal syndrome[a]	AKI in patient with decompensated chronic liver disease
A	Atheroembolism[a]	Triad of sub-acute renal failure, precipitating factor & purple toes
R	Renovascular[a]	Cardio-renal failure especially if hypertensive with asymmetrical kidney size
	Rhabdomyolysis[a]	Check CK if AKI with raised transaminases (AST > ALT) & normal bilirubin
M	Myeloma[a]	AKI in elderly if with anaemia, hypercalcaemia, back pain
	Malignant hypertension[a]	Severe HT with bilateral retinal haemorrhages and exudates and/or papilloedema
A	Acute on chronic	Previous SCr >150 μmol/L and/or bilateral small kidneys on sonar
C	CKD presenting acutely	Bilateral small kidneys, no previous bloods & no obvious reversible factors.

10.1 Causes of Acute Kidney Injury

Q1 What is meant by the term acute kidney injury?

Q2 Give a clinical approach to the diagnosis of unexplained renal failure.

Q3 How can you tell if AKI is acute or acute on chronic?

Q4 What is meant by chronic presenting acutely?

Q5 What do you understand by the term acute tubular necrosis (ATN)?

Q6 What are the four main risk factors for acute tubular necrosis?

Q7 Give ten important nephrotoxins.

Q8 How do ACEI and ARBs cause AKI?

Q9 How do NSAIDs cause AKI?

Q10 Who is most at risk of contrast nephropathy?

Q11 What steps might you take to prevent contrast nephropathy?

Q12 Explain why ciclosporin & tacrolimus – two drugs commonly used in transplantation – are double edged swords

Q13 What clinical features might suggest obstructive uropathy was the cause of AKI?

Q14 How might clinical examination suggest a diagnosis of obstructive uropathy?

Q15 How is the diagnosis of obstructive uropathy usually confirmed?

Q16 What are the causes of renal inflammation and what clues may there be that this is present?

Q17 What are the other important causes of AKI and describe how you might recognise these?

Further Reading

1. Lewington A, Kanagasundaram S. Acute Kidney Injury. Clinical Practice Guidelines, 5th edition. UK Renal Association, 2011. www.renal.org/guidelines/modules/acute-kidney-injury.

Rhabdomyolysis

11

Q1 What is rhabdomyolysis and how does it present?

The term rhabdomyolysis describes skeletal muscle breakdown regardless of the underlying cause. Clinical presentations range from an asymptomatic incidental finding on blood or urine testing, to muscle aches with dark coloured urine (myoglobin) through to a severe illness involving AKI requiring renal replacement therapy. The frequency of AKI in rhabdomyolysis is variable, being reported at 15–50 %.

Q2 What are the causes of rhabdomyolysis?

A recent review identified three physical and six non-physical causes. The physical causes are direct muscle injury, exertion or ischaemia. The non-physical causes comprise a diverse group of conditions including temperature extremes, electrolyte abnormalities, auto-immune disease, infections, drugs and toxins. Figure 11.1 shows the causes of rhabdomyolysis in a consecutive series of 92 patients with CK >10,000 iu/L in south west Scotland.

Q3 How does rhabdomyolysis lead to AKI?

Large quantities of electrolytes, enzymes and protein (myoglobin) are released into the circulation following damage to skeletal muscle. Myoglobin is thought to be the main culprit, leading to AKI by intra-tubular cast formation and a direct cytotoxic effect, though it does not do so in every case. Some patients have very high levels of CK in their serum and do not succumb to AKI. It seems likely that both hypovolaemia and aciduria must be present for AKI to occur.

Q4 What clinical clues would make you consider rhabdomyolysis?

There are usually a few clinical pointers towards this diagnosis. The history may reveal a period of immobility due to frailty or decreased conscious level – usually in the context of drug or alcohol use. A recent infective history, the addition of a new drug likely to cause or interact with current medication to cause rhabdomyolysis or strenuous unaccustomed exercise (e.g. marathon running) should always prompt the clinician to look for evidence of muscle damage. Visibly dark urine ("coke-coloured") is likely to be caused by myoglobinuria in the context of a compatible history. Incidentally, myoglobinuria will test positive for blood on the urine dipstick test without there being any red blood cells on microscopy

The cause of rhabdomyolysis in the following case history was a previously unsuspected drug interaction between atorvastatin and fusidic acid, diagnosed on the basis of muscle weakness and grossly raised CK. The patient was oligoanuric at the time so that it was not possible to test for myoglobinuria.

M. Findlay, C. Isles, *Clinical Companion in Nephrology*,
DOI 10.1007/978-3-319-14868-7_11, © Springer International Publishing Switzerland 2015

Fig. 11.1 Causes of rhabdomyolysis in 92 consecutive patients with serum CK >10,000 iu/l (Unpublished observations)

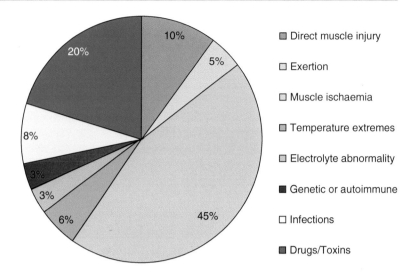

□ Direct muscle injury

□ Exertion

□ Muscle ischaemia

□ Temperature extremes

□ Electrolyte abnormality

■ Genetic or autoimmune

□ Infections

■ Drugs/Toxins

Case Report

A 69 year old man presented with multi organ failure secondary to left lower lobe consolidation for which he required ventilation, dialysis and inotropic support. One week previously he had been prescribed flucloxacillin 2 g per day and fusidic acid 2.25 g per day following the excision of an infected hip prosthesis. He had a myocardial infarction previously and his routine medications included atorvastatin 40 mg per day. We were able to withdraw ventilatory and circulatory support after 3 days, although the patient remained dialysis dependent and slow to mobilise. We observed at this point that he could not sit up unaided and went on to demonstrate proximal muscle weakness with serum CK 21,652 iu/l (normal range 0–195). Both atorvastatin and fusidic acid were stopped. The patient was unable to walk for a further 4 days and remained dialysis dependent for another 10 days. When reviewed at the clinic 2 months after his initial presentation muscle power had returned to normal and serum creatinine was 105 μmol/l.

Teckchandani, et al. Rhabdomyolysis following co-prescription of fusidic acid and atorvastatin. *J R Coll Phys Edinb*. 2010;40:33–6; with kind permission of the Royal College of Physicians of Edinburgh

Q5   Is the risk of rhabdomyolysis the same with all statins?

No. Statins are an important non-physical cause of rhabdomyolysis particularly when prescribed with drugs that interfere with their metabolism. The risk of rhabdomyolysis varies with the extent an individual statin is dependent for its metabolism on cytochrome P450 and the degree to which this enzyme's activity is inhibited by a particular antimicrobial as shown in the table below. The risk of rhabdomyolysis with simvastatin and clarithromycin is particularly important because patients with exacerbation of COPD and pneumonia who happen to be taking simvastatin are frequently given clarithromycin following admission to hospital. The case history described above suggests a further adverse interaction, this time between atorvastatin and fusidic acid (Fig. 11.2).

Q6   What biochemical clues would make you consider rhabdomyolysis?

Serum CK is not part of the routine biochemical blood screen which means that a diagnosis of rhabdomyolysis may be missed unless specifically considered. Fortunately, there may be other clues. Skeletal muscle also contains AST, ALT, LDH, aldolase, potassium, phosphate and uric acid. Elevated transaminases with normal bilirubin in a patient with unexplained AKI make a diagnosis of rhabdomyolysis worth considering and should prompt a request for serum CK. Serum AST will always be greater than serum ALT

Fig. 11.2 Statins and risk of rhabdomyolysis (Reproduced by kind permission © 2010 Royal College of Physicians Edinburgh. *J R Coll Physicians Edinb.* 2010;40:33–6)

	Prava	Fluva	Simva	Atorva	Rosuva
	Not by p450	Mainly 2C9, partly 2C8, 3A4	Mainly 3A4	Partly 3A4	<10% by 2C9, 2C19
Clarithro 3A4	Caution	Should be safe	Omit	Omit or Max 20mg	Should be safe
Erythro 3A4	Caution	Should be safe	Omit	Omit or Max 10mg	Should be safe

when rhabdomyolysis is present – another important clue to diagnosis.

Q7   How do you confirm rhabdomyolysis?

A diagnosis of rhabdomyolysis is not always as easy to establish as it ought to be. The triad of muscle pain and/or weakness with myoglobinuria and elevated creatinine kinase (CK) is diagnostic, but muscle pain/weakness is present in only 50 % of cases while myoglobinuria has a short half-life of only 2–3 h and is detected in only 20 % of cases. Furthermore, there is no agreed diagnostic cut-point for serum CK – some say five or ten times upper limit of the normal range of 0–195 iu/l, others greater than 5,000 iu/l or greater than 10,000 iu/l (Fig. 11.3).

Q8   What is Compartment Syndrome and how might this be treated?

Compartment syndrome can be both a cause and a complication of rhabdomyolysis. Crush injuries may cause the affected muscles to swell while muscles damaged by one of the non-physical causes may swell too. Muscles in the forearm, lower leg and some other body areas are surrounded by fibrous bands, creating distinct compartments. These fibrous bands cannot stretch to accommodate the swollen muscles, leading to irreversible nerve and muscle injury if the swelling is left untreated. Surgical fasciotomy may then be indicated. It is important therefore to examine patients thor-

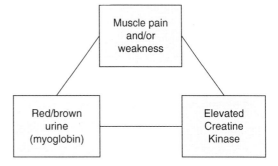

Fig. 11.3 Diagnostic triad for rhabdomyolysis

oughly and consider compartment syndrome in all patients with rhabdomyolysis.

Q9   How would you manage a patient with rhabdomyolysis?

Patients with rhabdomyolysis are usually volume deplete due to sequestration of water in damaged muscle and because of this volume repletion is the mainstay of therapy. Some recommend alkalinisation of urine because myoglobin is more likely to precipitate in the renal tubules when urine is acidic, though randomised trials of alkalinisation have failed to establish benefit. Hyperkalaemia is more likely to occur than in other forms of AKI because potassium is released from damaged muscles, and should be treated accordingly (see Chap. 18). The indications for dialysis in rhabdomyolysis induced AKI are the same as for other forms of AKI.

11.1   Objectives: Rhabdomyolysis

After reading this chapter, you should be able to answer the following:

Q1   **What is rhabdomyolysis and how does it present?**

Q2   **What are the causes of rhabdomyolysis?**

Q3   **How does rhabdomyolysis lead to AKI?**

Q4   **What clinical clues would make you consider rhabdomyolysis?**

Q5   **Is the risk of rhabdomyolysis the same with all statins?**

Q6   **What biochemical clues would make you consider rhabdomyolysis?**

Q7   **How do you confirm rhabdomyolysis?**

Q8   **What is Compartment Syndrome and how might this be treated?**

Q9   **How would you manage a patient with rhabdomyolysis?**

Further Reading

1. Bosch X, et al. Rhabdomyolysis and acute kidney injury. N Engl J Med. 2009;361:62–72.

Cardiorenal Failure

Q1 What is meant by the term cardiorenal failure?

Originally this was a term used to describe declining renal function in patients with advanced heart failure. Subsequently it was defined as a 'pathophysiological disorder in which acute or chronic dysfunction of one organ may induce acute or chronic dysfunction in the other'. From a clinical point of view cardiorenal failure is best thought of as any disorder in which cardiac and renal dysfunction coexist.

Q2 Why is cardiorenal failure important?

Cardiorenal failure is common. In a large US registry based study, 9 % of patients with new onset heart failure or decompensated chronic established HF whose symptoms were sufficient to warrant hospitalisation had serum creatinine >265 umol/l. Cardiorenal failure is also dangerous. In a study of 1,004 patients hospitalized with symptoms and signs of heart failure, 27 % developed worsening renal function. There was a sevenfold increased risk of death in hospital in this group, after adjusting for medical history, clinical signs and lab values. From a practical point of view, it is not generally possible to treat the pulmonary congestion of cardiorenal failure with a bigger dose of diuretic without aggravating the renal failure.

Q3 What are the causes of cardiorenal failure?

The classification of causes adopted by experts in this field recognises five subtypes: acute or chronic cardiorenal, acute or chronic renocardiac and a fifth group in which systemic diseases such as sepsis cause both. This is not a clinician friendly classification as it makes little or no mention of the only potentially 'curable' cause of cardiorenal failure, namely bilateral renovascular disease, and also does not acknowledge the confounding influence of ACEI/ARBs. A more practical approach is to consider that either the heart causes the kidneys to fail, that the kidneys cause the heart to fail, something else causes both or the two are unrelated. These four diagnostic categories are described in more detail in the box.

Box 12.1 Causes of Cardiorenal Failure
- **Cardiac disease causes the renal failure.** In an inpatient setting the classic presentation is a result of cardiogenic shock. In the outpatient clinic it is more likely to be a consequence of an ACE inhibitor or angiotensin receptor blocker
- **Renal disease causes the cardiac failure.** This most often occurs when a dialysis patient fails to comply with fluid restriction & presents with shortness of breath due to fluid overload.
- **Bilateral renovascular disease causes both cardiac & renal failure.** This is the most interesting of the causes because it offers the chance of a cure for both the

---

M. Findlay, C. Isles, *Clinical Companion in Nephrology*,
DOI 10.1007/978-3-319-14868-7_12, © Springer International Publishing Switzerland 2015

cardiac & the renal failure. Unfortunately, reversible cardiorenal failure due to bilateral renovascular disease only accounts for a small proportion of patients who present in this way. The others have hypertensive nephrosclerosis.

- **Unrelated aetiology.** One disease e.g. myocardial infarction causes the cardiac failure and another unrelated disease e.g. glomerulonephritis causes the renal failure.

Q4   When might you suspect bilateral renovascular disease as a cause of cardiorenal failure?

All patients with cardiorenal failure should have echo and renal ultrasound as part of their initial investigations. An echo showing LVH without dilatation (Fig. 12.1) and a renal ultrasound showing inequality of renal size (one kidney ≥1.5 cm smaller than the other) is highly suggestive, although it should be borne in mind that patients with bilateral renovascular disease do not always have significant asymmetry. Acute renal deterioration following ACE inhibitor is another useful clue (see case history and Fig. 12.2). In cases where revascularisation would be appropriate these findings should lead to imaging of the renal arteries (see Q7, Chap. 23).

Case Report

A 75 year old woman with previous inferior myocardial infarction required temporary haemodialysis when she became moribund with cardiorenal failure while receiving an angiotensin converting enzyme inhibitor. Blood pressure was 102/58 mmHg and she had gross pulmonary and peripheral oedema. Echo showed LVH. Her serum creatinine concentration was 731 μmol/l. She had had three less severe episodes of cardiorenal failure in the previous 15 months, each associated with an angiotensin converting enzyme inhibitor. The left kidney measured 7.0 cm on ultrasonography and the right kidney 9.5 cm. Arteriography showed occlusion of the left renal artery and 90 % stenosis of the right renal artery, which was stented. An angiotensin converting enzyme inhibitor was restarted. During 8 months follow up (see below) she had no further episodes of cardiac or renal failure. Blood pressure at her last visit was 193/81 mmHg and a serum creatinine concentration was 110 μmol/l while taking lisinopril 20 mg daily, frusemide 20 mg daily, amlodipine 10 mg daily, simvastatin 20 mg at night and aspirin 75 mg daily.

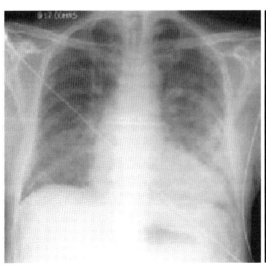 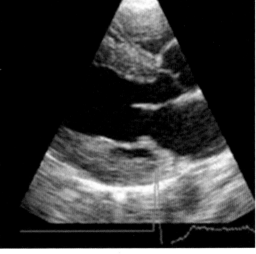

Fig. 12.1   Chest X-ray appearance of pulmonary oedema with cardiomegaly (*left*) and cardiac ECHO showing LVH without LV dilation

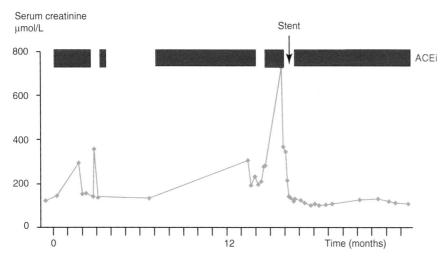

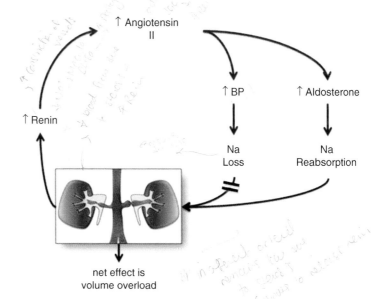

Fig. 12.2 Serum creatinine plotted against time in the patient whose case history is described above. Note marked rise in serum creatinine with ACEI which did not recur following renal artery stent insertion (Reproduced from Brammah A, et al. Bilateral renovascular disease causing cardiorenal failure. *BMJ*. 2003;326:489–91; with permission from BMJ Publishing Group Ltd)

Fig. 12.3 Mechanism of volume overload in patients with renovascular disease

Q5   Why do patients with bilateral renovascular disease develop cardiac failure?

The mechanism of the cardiac failure in bilateral renovascular disease is shown in the figure. Essentially this is a consequence of fluid retention due to the unopposed action of aldosterone. Sodium loss (via pressure natriuresis) does not occur because the kidneys do not sense the high blood pressure as they are protected by their narrowed renal arteries (Fig. 12.3).

Q6   What is the preferred method of revascularisation?

Historically, this was by aorto-renal bypass, a major surgical undertaking. The number of patients being put forward for intervention increased with the advent of angioplasty, though elastic recoil of ostial stenoses meant that this was not always technically successful. The preferred method of renal artery revascularisation, when it is agreed that this should be undertaken,

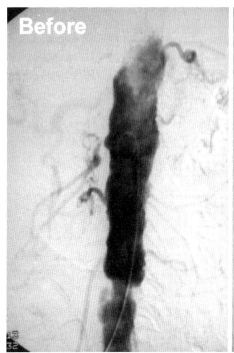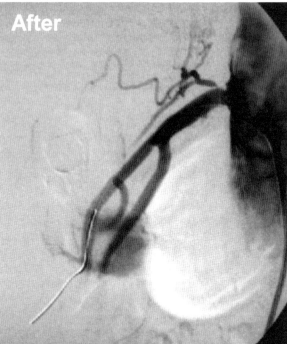

Fig. 12.4 Renal angiogram showing atheromatous aorta, left renal artery occlusion and tight right renal artery stenosis (*before*); & right renal artery guidewire with stent (*after*) (Reproduced from Brammah A, et al. Bilateral renovascular disease causing cardiorenal failure. *BMJ*. 2003;326:489–91; with permission from BMJ Publishing Group Ltd)

is now percutaneous transluminal renal angioplasty with stent (Fig. 12.4).

Q7 How should you manage cardiorenal failure in hospital in patients who do not have bilateral renovascular disease?

This is a common clinical scenario. For patients admitted as an emergency with cardiorenal failure in whom the cardiac failure predominates, you can try frusemide IV with salt and water restriction, while recognising that worsening kidney function may be the price you have to pay in order to keep lungs free of fluid. If renal failure predominates a cautious trial of fluid is indicated, while recognising that peripheral oedema may be an acceptable compromise in the trade-off between heart and kidneys. This is usually tricky, often requires senior help and sometimes dialysis or haemofiltration.

Q8 Should patients with cardiorenal failure be offered an ACE inhibitor or ARB?

Patients with cardiorenal failure are also frequently encountered in clinics where the question of treatment with ACEI/ARB invariably arises. Renal function may improve, stay the same or deteriorate with these drugs and often the only way to find out is to prescribe and see what happens. A modest rise in creatinine of less than 30 % or fall in GFR of less than <25 % with ACEI/ARB is usually considered an acceptable price to be paid for keeping the lungs free of fluid. It is generally advised that these drugs are not started if serum K is greater than 5 mmol/l and that they are withdrawn if serum K exceeds 6 mmol/l during treatment and other drugs that may cause hyperkalemia have been stopped. Substitution of the ACEI/ARB by hydralazine/nitrate, a combination of arterial and venous vasodilator which has been shown to improve symptoms but not prognosis in heart failure, can be considered if serum K, serum creatinine and/or GFR preclude treatment with drugs that block the renin-angiotensin system.

12.1 Objectives: Cardiorenal Failure

After reading this chapter you should be able to answer the following:

Q1 What is meant by the term cardiorenal failure?

Q2 Why is cardiorenal failure important?

Q3 What are the causes of cardiorenal failure?

Q4 When might you suspect bilateral renovascular disease as a cause of cardiorenal failure?

Q5 Why do patients with bilateral renovascular disease develop cardiac failure?

Q6 What is the preferred method of revascularisation?

Q7 How should you manage cardiorenal failure in hospital in patients who do not have bilateral renovascular disease?

Q8 Should patients with cardiorenal failure be offered an ACE inhibitor or ARB?

Further Reading

1. Ronco C, et al. Cardio-renal syndromes: report from the consensus conference of the Acute Dialysis Quality Initiative. Eur Heart J. 2010;31:703–11.

Q1 What is hepatorenal syndrome?

Hepatorenal syndrome (HRS) is defined as the occurrence of renal failure in a patient with advanced liver disease in the absence of an identifiable cause of renal failure. It is a diagnosis of exclusion. More commonly a complication of chronic liver disease, HRS will develop in up to 40 % of patients with advanced cirrhosis and ascites by 5 years. HRS can also complicate acute liver failure in those who present with fulminant hepatic failure of any cause (e.g. severe alcoholic or viral hepatitis).

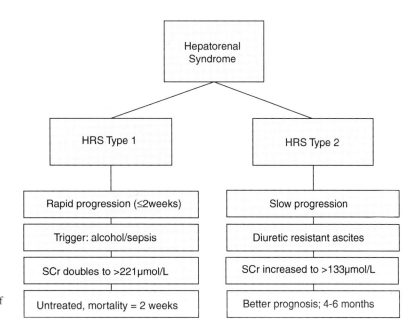

Fig. 13.1 The two types of hepatorenal syndrome

M. Findlay, C. Isles, *Clinical Companion in Nephrology*,
DOI 10.1007/978-3-319-14868-7_13, © Springer International Publishing Switzerland 2015

Q2 There are two types of HRS. Discuss.

Type 1 HRS is characterised by doubling of serum creatinine to a final value greater than 221 μmol/l over a period of less than 2 weeks. It is usually triggered by an episode of severe alcoholic hepatitis or by a septic insult such as spontaneous bacterial peritonitis (SBP) in a patient with end stage liver disease. Untreated the median survival of type 1 HRS is approximately 2 weeks.

Type 2 HRS occurs in patients with diuretic resistant ascites. It is characterised by a slower and less progressive rise in serum creatinine to a value exceeding 133 μmol/l. It carries a better prognosis than type 1 HRS with a median survival of 4–6 months (Fig. 13.1).

Q3 Describe the pathophysiology of HRS.

This is complex. There are at least three key features: Splanchnic vasodilatation in response to nitric oxide produced as a result of decreased hepatic perfusion; impairment of cardiac function due to cirrhotic cardiomyopathy and reduced production of renal prostaglandins which normally dilate the afferent arteriole. All three mechanisms will compromise renal perfusion.

Q4 How do you diagnose HRS?

There is no single diagnostic test. Rather HRS is deemed likely in a patient with clinical stigmata of cirrhosis who develops acute kidney injury (type 1) or more slowly progressive renal failure (type 2) in the absence of other obvious causes of acute kidney injury. Diuretic resistant ascites may or may not be present in type 1 and is always present in type 2. Previously, on-going bacterial infection excluded HRS but it is now recognised that bacterial infection and in particular SBP is the most important trigger. The revised International Ascites Club criteria for HRS are shown in the box.

Box 13.1 Criteria for Diagnosis of Hepatorenal Syndrome in Cirrhosis

- Cirrhosis with ascites.
- Serum creatinine >133 μmol/l.
- Absence of shock
- Absence of hypovolaemia as defined by no sustained improvement of renal function (creatinine decreasing to <133 μmol/l) following at least 2 days of diuretic withdrawal (if on diuretics) and volume expansion with albumin at 1 g/kg/day up to a maximum of 100 g/day.
- No current or recent treatment with nephrotoxic drugs.
- Absence of parenchymal renal disease as defined by urine PCR <50 mg/mmol, no visible or non-visible haematuria, and normal renal ultrasound

Q5 What general measures are of value in HRS?

Patients with HRS type 1 should be admitted to a high dependency unit for supportive care. Intravascular volume expansion is important but often difficult to judge as excessive IV fluid may lead to worsening of ascites, pleural effusion, heart failure and dilutional hyponatraemia. All diuretics should be stopped, at least initially, and potassium sparing diuretics should be avoided because of the risk of life threatening hyperkalaemia. Precipitating factors such as SBP should be sought and treated if present. Large volume paracentesis is indicated in patients with tense ascites, with intravenous albumin replacement (by infusing 8 g albumin/l of ascitic fluid removed) to maintain ECF homeostasis. There are no data to say whether it is better to stop or continue beta-blockers in patients who are taking these drugs to prevent variceal bleeding.

Q6 What specific drug therapy has been found to be of value in HRS?

Terlipressin, a vasopressin analogue that vasoconstricts the splanchnic vascular bed, improves renal function in 40–50 % of patients with type 1 HRS. It is usually given in combination with albumin. The doses of both drugs are shown in the box.

Box 13.2 Terlipressin and Albumin for HRS

- Rx terlipressin at 1 mg qds increasing to 2 mg qds if serum creatinine does not fall by at least 25 % by day 3 of therapy.
- Maintain treatment until serum creatinine has fallen below 133 µmol/l. Median time to response is 14 days.
- Terlipressin is contraindicated in patients with ischaemic vascular diseases and signs of splanchnic or digital ischaemia.
- Recurrence after withdrawal of therapy is uncommon and re-treatment with terlipressin is generally effective
- In most studies terlipressin was given with albumin 1 g/kg on day 1 followed by 20–40 g/day to improve the efficacy of treatment on circulatory function

---

Q7 What is the role of renal replacement therapy in HRS?

The indications for RRT in HRS are the same as the indications for RRT in patients with other causes of acute kidney injury i.e. uraemia, overload, hyperkalaemia, pericarditis and acidosis. RRT is not a first-line treatment in HRS because it does not correct the underlying problem though

it can tide the patient over until the liver recovers or be employed as a bridge to liver transplantation. Both intermittent haemodialysis and continuous haemofiltration have been used with no evidence to suggest that one is superior to the other.

Q8 What other non-pharmacological treatments may have a role in the management of HRS?

These are transjugular intrahepatic portosystemic shunts (TIPS) and liver transplantation. Correcting portal hypertension by TIPS has been reported to improve renal function in some patients but the risk of encephalopathy means that the procedure is often contraindicated. Liver transplantation is the definitive treatment for both type 1 and type 2 HRS. HRS should be treated pharmacologically before liver transplantation because this improves post-liver transplant outcomes. The kidneys generally recover following successful liver transplantation.

Q9 Can hepatorenal syndrome be prevented?

The treatment of SBP with broad spectrum antibiotic such as co-amoxiclav or ceftriaxone and an intravenous albumin infusion reduces the risk of developing HRS in patients with SBP. Long term oral administration of norfloxacin 400 mg per day in patients with advanced cirrhosis has also been shown to reduce the risk of HRS and improve survival.

Q10 What is the outcome of hepatorenal syndrome?

Poor. As a general rule the kidneys don't improve until the liver improves and unless there is an obvious trigger such as SBP the liver very often doesn't. Untreated, most patients will die within 2–4 weeks from the start of their renal decline. Terlipressin and albumin have improved the outlook for patients with HRS but only around 50 % respond to therapy.

13.1 Objectives: Hepatorenal Syndrome

Q1 What is hepatorenal syndrome?

Q2 There are two types of HRS. Discuss.

Q3 Describe the pathophysiology of HRS.

Q4 How do you diagnose HRS?

Q5 What general measures are of value in HRS?

Q6 What specific drug therapy has been found to be of value in HRS?

Q7 What is the role of renal replacement therapy in HRS?

Q8 What other non-pharmacological treatments may have a role in the management of HRS?

Q9 Can hepatorenal syndrome be prevented?

Q10 What is the outcome of hepatorenal syndrome?

Further Reading

1. Davenport A, et al. Medical management of hepatorenal syndrome. Nephrol Dial Transplant. 2012;27: 34–41.
2. European Association for Study of the Liver. EASL clinical practice guidelines on the management of ascites, spontaneous bacterial peritonitis, and hepatorenal syndrome in cirrhosis. J Hepatol. 2010;53:397–417.

Q1 What does the abbreviation HUS/TTP stand for?

It stands for Haemolytic Uraemic Syndrome/ Thrombotic Thrombocytopenic Purpura, two clinical syndromes each characterized by Microangiopathic Haemolytic Anaemia (MAHA) and thrombocytopenia. The term thrombotic microangiopathy is used to describe patients with these disorders. Although there are subtle differences between HUS and TTP (see Q7), it is helpful to consider them as different manifestations of the same disease process

Q2 What is meant by the term Microangiopathic Haemolytic Anaemia?

MAHA is a sine qua non of HUS/TTP. It is a form of intravascular haemolysis with prominent red cell fragmentation (schistocytes) on the blood film. Red cells fragment when they are caught on fibrin strands in the microcirculation (Fig. 14.1).

Q3 What other features of haemolysis will be present in these patients?

The haemolysis of MAHA is typically associated with evidence of intravascular red cell destruction (raised indirect bilirubin, reduced serum haptoglobin) and compensatory increased red cell production (raised reticulocyte count). Serum LDH is usually extremely high reflecting both haemolysis and tissue damage due to systemic ischaemia. Because the haemolysis is non-immune the direct Coomb's test (direct antibody test) will be negative.

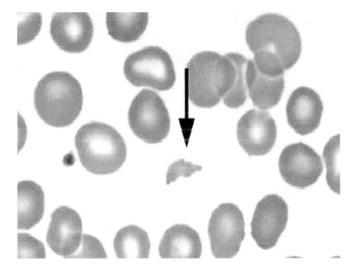

Fig. 14.1 Schistocyte (*arrowed*) as seen on a blood film

M. Findlay, C. Isles, *Clinical Companion in Nephrology*,
DOI 10.1007/978-3-319-14868-7_14, © Springer International Publishing Switzerland 2015

Q4   What is the commonest cause of HUS/TTP in adults?

Most cases are in adults are due to ADAMTS13 deficiency which may be congenital or required. ADAMTS13 is a specific von Willebrand factor (vWF) cleaving enzyme. Congenital cases are usually due to inherited deficiency while acquired cases are more likely a consequence of an auto-antibody to this enzyme.

Q5   How does ADAMTS13 deficiency cause HUS/TTP?

Healthy endothelial cells produce vWF – a protein that is unfolded by shear stresses in the circulation then cleaved by a metalloproteinase enzyme called ADAMTS13 in order to support platelet adhesion (Fig. 14.2).

Absence or reduced activity of the vWF cleaving enzyme leads to a build-up of unusually large vWF molecules which in turn cause platelet aggregation in the microcirculation, so called Thrombotic Microangiopathy (TMA) (Fig. 14.3)

Q6   What other causes of adult HUS/TTP are there?

Adult HUS/TTP may also be caused by Shiga Toxin producing E Coli (STEC-HUS) diarrhoea which is the commonest cause in children; drugs

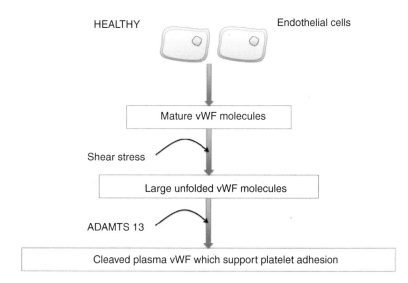

Fig. 14.2 Normal mechanism of ADAMTS13 cleaving vWF molecules to support normal platelet adhesion

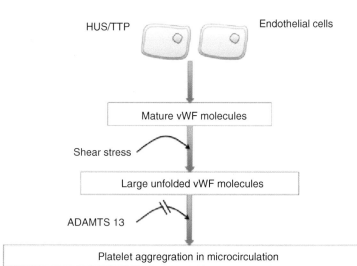

Fig. 14.3 Absence of ADAMTS13 results in persistence of large vWF molecules triggering abnormal platelet aggregation in the microcirculation

esp. quinine, the calcineurin inhibitors cyclosporin and tacrolimus, and some cancer drugs esp. gemcitabine; and pregnancy in which it may be difficult to distinguish HUS/TTP from severe preeclampsia and the HELLP syndrome. Below is a case of TTP triggered by infection with the gram negative rod, capnocytophaga canimorsus.

Case Report

A 53 year old woman presented with septicaemia due to capnocytophaga canimorsus, an organism that is known to produce a wide spectrum of disease following dog bites. She subsequently became confused and developed multi organ failure with mottled peripheries leading to frank gangrenous changes affecting all the toes and haemorrhagic ulceration of the nose and mouth. Her platelet count fell to 27,000/mm^2 in association with red cell fragments on her blood film, although the rest of her clotting screen was essentially normal. These findings led us to consider a diagnosis of thrombotic thrombocytopenic purpura, following which her treatment was modified to include plasma exchange and high dose steroids. She went on to require 16 days of plasma exchange and 32 days of haemofiltration before her renal function recovered. Her improvement thereafter

was sustained though she required partial amputation of several toes and plastic surgery to her nose. Blood urea on discharge from hospital 6 weeks after admission was 5.4 mmol/l with serum creatinine 111 μmol/l.

Finn M, et al. Beware of the dog! A syndrome resembling thrombotic thrombocytopenic purpura associated with Capnocytophaga canimorsus septicaemia. *Nephrol Dial Transplant* 1996;11: 1839–40; with permission from Oxford University Press

Q7   How is a diagnosis of HUS/TTP usually established?

HUS/TTP may be thought of as a pentad comprising MAHA and thrombocytopenia in all cases, together with AKI, neurological abnormalities and cardiac disease in some. If AKI is present the disorder is more likely to be HUS whereas if neurological abnormalities predominate then the term TTP may be preferred. The distinction is probably a little artificial. Neurological symptoms usually fluctuate and range from confusion and headache through TIA and stroke to seizures and coma. Cardiac involvement may be present in up to 20 % patients and manifest by arrhythmia, MI, sudden cardiac death and heart failure. High fever with rigors suggests sepsis rather than HUS/TTP (Fig. 14.4).

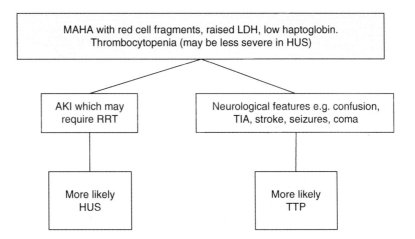

Fig. 14.4 Summary of differences between HUS and TTP

Q8   Red cell fragments may be seen in other conditions. Discuss.

MAHA with red cell fragments may be a feature of malignant hypertension (MHT), scleroderma renal crisis and DIC. The distinction is important because treatment differs. Patients with MHT will generally have diastolic pressure ≥ 130 mmHg with bilateral retinal haemorrhages and soft exudates. The presence of sclerodactyly and Raynaud's phenomenon together with specific auto antibodies e.g. anti-centromere and anti-Scl 70 will favour a diagnosis of progressive systemic sclerosis, while DIC is characterized by an abnormal clotting screen with raised PT/APTT in addition to low fibrinogen (the clotting screen in HUS/TTP should be normal).

Q9   How would you treat an adult patient with HUS/TTP?

The cornerstone of management is plasma exchange which should be started as soon as possible in order to reduce the otherwise very high mortality associated with HUS/TTP. The recommendation to use plasma exchange extends to adult STEC-HUS though the evidence base for this advice is not as strong as for patients with ADAMTS13 deficiency. Plasma exchange with fresh frozen plasma (or in some units Octaplas, a form of FFP treated to reduce the risk of transmitting blood borne viruses) removes the abnormal vWF molecules and the ADAMTS13 autoantibody, while replacing the missing enzyme. Daily plasma exchange is recommended until the platelet count and LDH return to normal. See Appendix 6 for more details.

Q10   When might you give steroids?

Steroids are widely used in combination with plasma exchange in the treatment of auto-immune TTP in adults. Evidence supports their use particularly in patients whose platelet counts do not begin to rise after several days of plasma exchange and in those whose thrombocytopenia recurs after PE has been discontinued. The recommended dose is 1 mg/kg of oral prednisolone. By contrast, STEC- HUS in children usually remits with supportive care, although over half of affected children may require renal dialysis.

Q11   What is the outcome of adult HUS/TTP?

Idiopathic HUS/TTP is a medical emergency with high mortality of up to 90 % unless treated effectively and promptly. Mortality with plasma exchange is still around 20 %. Survivors may have residual cognitive defects and/or incomplete recovery of their renal function.

14.1   Objectives: HUS/TTP in Adults

Q1   What does the abbreviation HUS/TTP stand for?

Q2   What is meant by the term Microangiopathic Haemolytic Anaemia?

Q3   What other features of haemolysis will be present in these patients?

Q4   What is the commonest cause of HUS/TTP in adults?

Q5   How does ADAMTS13 deficiency cause HUS/TTP?

Q6   What other causes of adult HUS/TTP are there?

Q7   How is a diagnosis of HUS/TTP usually established?

Q8   Red cell fragments may be seen in other conditions. Discuss.

Q9   How would you treat an adult patient with HUS/TTP?

Q10   When might you give steroids?

Q11   What is the outcome of adult HUS/TTP?

Further Reading

1. Scully M, Hunt BJ, Benjamin S, Liesner R, Rose P, Peyvandi F, Cheung B, and Machin SJ, British Committee for Standards in Haematology. Guidelines on the diagnosis and management of thrombotic thrombocytopenic purpura and other thrombotic microangiopathies. Br J Haematol. 2012;158(3):323–35.

Q1   What are plasma cells and what do they normally do?

Plasma cells are terminally differentiated B lymphocytes that produce large amounts of specific immunoglobulin. Immunoglobulins are the antibodies that make up part of our host defences. The immunoglobulins produced in health are polyclonal i.e. a mixture of IgG, IgA and IgM heavy chains with kappa and lambda light chains. Kappa and lambda light chains are not always attached to their heavy chains in which case they are known as free light chains (FLC).

Q2   What is myeloma?

Myeloma (sometimes known as multiple myeloma) is a malignant tumour of plasma cells producing immunoglobulins. Whereas normal immunoglobulin production is polyclonal (see above) the immunoglobulins produced in myeloma are monoclonal meaning that they derive from an abnormal clone of plasma cells (essentially a single plasma cell that becomes malignant and begins to multiply). This monoclonal protein is sometimes referred to as a paraprotein. Myeloma accounts for 1 % of all cancers and is the second most common haematological malignancy after non-Hodgkin's lymphomas (Fig. 15.1).

Q3   Do all patients with myeloma produce monoclonal proteins?

Over 95 % do. Around 55 % of myelomas are known as IgG myeloma because the heavy chain class is IgG. Twenty percent are IgA myeloma for the same reason. IgG and IgA myelomas are usually associated with increased serum FLC which are either kappa or lambda but not both. When the serum FLC production rate exceeds the reabsorptive capacity of the renal tubules then the FLC are detectable in the urine as Bence Jones proteins. Around 10 % of patients with myeloma produce FLC only (aka Light Chain myeloma, previously known as Bence Jones myeloma). An IgM monoclonal protein usually means that the patient has a lymphoma (see later). IgD and IgE myelomas are extremely rare as are myelomas in patients who do not secrete immunoglobulins, so-called non-secretory myelomas.

Q4   How does myeloma present clinically?

Myeloma is a haematological disorder that frequently presents to general physicians and nephrologists. Myeloma may be asymptomatic and only detected because a doctor acted on a clinical clue e.g. anaemia with high ESR. Alternatively it can present with symptoms. Haematologists regularly use the acronym CRAB as an aide-memoire: hyperCalcaemia, Renal injury, Anaemia and Bony lesions. Acute kidney injury requiring dialysis is a renal emergency. Back pain due to myeloma causing spinal cord compression is a potentially devastating complication of myeloma.

M. Findlay, C. Isles, *Clinical Companion in Nephrology*,
DOI 10.1007/978-3-319-14868-7_15, © Springer International Publishing Switzerland 2015

Fig. 15.1 Plasma cells and immunoglobulins

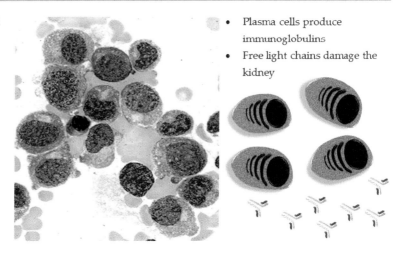

- Plasma cells produce immunoglobulins
- Free light chains damage the kidney

Q5 What might lead you to suspect that myeloma was the cause of the renal failure?

There will usually be some clues. The important ones are as follows:

- Anaemia with ESR >100.
- Hypercalcaemia – this is unusual in other causes of renal failure which are more commonly associated with hypocalcaemia.
- Serum total protein >100 g/l – if serum albumin is normal then this implies an excess of globulins and should prompt a request for serum electrophoresis.
- Bone pain e.g. back pain.

Q6 How would you confirm a diagnosis of myeloma?

This requires at least two of the following three features to be present:

- Monoclonal protein in serum and/or urine – usually IgG greater than 30 g/l or IgA greater than 20 g/l but there is no minimum level that excludes the diagnosis. Immune paresis i.e. suppression of the other immunoglobulin classes is commonly present.
- Presence of clonal plasma cells in bone marrow – usually greater than 10 % but no minimum level.
- Presence of myeloma related organ damage e.g. anaemia, lytic bone lesions, hypercalcaemia or kidney injury

We summarise the diagnostic criteria for myeloma in Fig. 15.2

Q7 How do we detect monoclonal proteins in serum and urine?

Traditionally, by requesting serum electrophoresis and urine for Bence Jones protein. Serum electrophoresis detects intact monoclonal immunoglobulin while Bence Jones proteins are free light chains that have spilled over into the urine. It is important to have some measure of free light chain production as 10 % of myelomas secrete free light chains rather than intact immunoglobulins (so called light chain or Bence Jones myeloma). Although not yet recommended as first line screening for myeloma, serum free light chains should be requested in patients in whom myeloma is felt likely but serum electrophoresis and urinary Bence Jones protein is negative. This is because FLC will be detectable before urinary BJP become positive (see Q8).

Q8 Why might serum free light chains be more useful than Bence Jones protein when diagnosing myeloma?

Serum FLC are filtered by the glomerulus and reabsorbed by the proximal tubules. The serum kappa/lambda ratio in health lies between 0.26 and 1.65. The kappa/lambda ratio in patients with renal disease has a wider range from 0.37 to 3.1, because renal impairment can reduce light chain

Fig. 15.2 Diagnosis of
myeloma

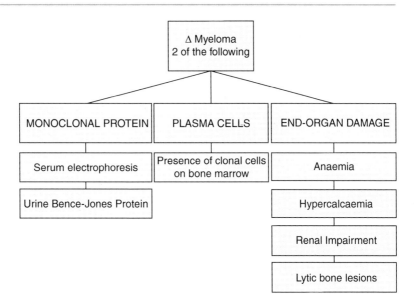

excretion. The reabsorptive capacity of the PCT (10–30 g/day) far exceeds the FLC production rate (0.5 g/day) which means that detection of urine FLC (Bence Jones protein) is a poor way of diagnosing myeloma, particularly if urine is dilute. Moreover, patients with oligo-anuric AKI may not pass enough urine to detect urine BJP. It is also surprising how often a urine sample for BJP is requested in hospital but not collected and so fails to arrive at the lab.

Q9 How does myeloma cause kidney injury?

Renal disease is almost always due to free light chains. When the concentration of clonal FLC in the glomerular filtrate exceeds the reabsorptive capacity of the proximal tubular epithelium, FLCs co-precipitate with Tamm-Horsfall protein in distal tubules to produce casts. In addition, clonal FLC have a direct inflammatory and cytotoxic effect on proximal tubular epithelium. The histological lesion is called cast nephropathy or myeloma kidney. The other causes for renal impairment in myeloma are drugs (chemo and NSAIDS), amyloid, volume depletion, hypercalcaemia, hyperuricemia and renal tubular dysfunction.

Q10 What are the treatment options for patients with myeloma?

The management of myeloma continues to evolve. High quality supportive care with optimisa-

tion of fluid balance, treatment of hypercalcaemia and avoidance of nephrotoxic drugs is very important. Biphosphonates e.g. zoledronate can reduce progression of bone disease by inhibiting osteoclastic activity. The mainstay of management in patients with renal failure is prompt and appropriate chemotherapy, usually with two drugs: high dose dexamethasone, and bortezomib, a proteosome inhibitor. For more detailed discussion of chemotherapy options see the latest British Committee for Standards in Haematology guidelines. This may be followed in younger patients by autologous (i.e. the patient's own) stem cell transplantation. Other treatment options include palliative care for the frail elderly and regular follow up without active treatment if there is no myeloma related organ damage or marrow impairment.

Q11 If the renal disease in myeloma is due to free light chains why not remove them by plasma exchange?

The role of extra-corporeal removal of FLC is currently unclear. Plasma exchange removes FLC but is probably ineffective because most FLC are extra-vascular. Using a high cut off dialyser which is particularly efficient at removing kappa and lambda light chains may improve outcomes. At present there is insufficient evidence to recommend the use of this technology in routine clinical practice.

Q12 What is the likely prognosis in myeloma?

It is not possible to cure myeloma in the same way that patients with lymphoma can be cured unless patients are suitable for allogeneic (i.e. someone else's) stem cell transplant and only a small proportion of younger patients are. Median survival with effective treatment for myeloma without kidney failure is now around 5 years and increasing year on year. By contrast, patients with myeloma who require dialysis and do not recover their renal function have considerably poorer outcomes.

Q13 What do you understand by the term monoclonal gammopathy of uncertain significance (MGUS)?

MGUS is the term used to describe patients who have a stable paraprotein in their serum (less commonly their urine) without evidence of associated disease. It is common and increases with age, affecting up to 5 % of the over 70 s. In a patient with MGUS the serum monoclonal IgG will usually be less than 30 g/l and the monoclonal IgA less than 20 g/l. There will usually be no Bence Jones protein in the urine and no immune-paresis. There will be no evidence of myeloma rated organ damage or marrow impairment by definition. These patients should have repeat serum and urine electrophoresis (or repeat serum electrophoresis and serum FLC depending on availability) every 6 months as there is a low but significant rate of transformation to myeloma of around 1 % per year.

Q14 What other plasma cell dyscrasias do you know?

Myeloma is most common. Patients with an IgM paraprotein invariably turn out to have a form of lymphoma. Waldenstrom's macroglobulinaemia is the most common of these, and may present with evidence of hyperviscosity syndrome e.g. headache, dizziness, vertigo, somnolence, confusion and ataxia. Cold agglutinin

disease is often due to an IgM paraprotein in a patient with a lymphoma. Primary amyloidosis shares many features with myeloma and should be suspected in a patient with a serum monoclonal protein and nephrotic range proteinuria. Tissue (e.g. a kidney biopsy) that stains pink with Congo red and shows characteristic apple-green birefringence on polarised light is required for a diagnosis. Treatment of primary amyloidosis is similar to the treatment of myeloma.

15.1   Myeloma and the Kidney

Q1   What are plasma cells and what do they normally do?

Q2   What is myeloma?

Q3   Do all patients with myeloma produce monoclonal proteins?

Q4   How does myeloma present clinically?

Q5   What might lead you to suspect that myeloma was the cause of the renal failure?

Q6   How would you confirm a diagnosis of myeloma?

Q7   How do we detect monoclonal proteins in serum and urine?

Q8   Why might serum free light chains be more useful than Bence Jones protein when diagnosing myeloma?

Q9   How does myeloma cause kidney injury?

Q10 What are the treatment options for patients with myeloma?

Q11 If the renal disease in myeloma is due to free light chains why not remove them by plasma exchange?

Q12 What is the likely prognosis in myeloma?

Q13 What do you understand by the term monoclonal gammopathy of uncertain significance (MGUS)?

Q14 What other plasma cell dyscrasias do you know?

Further Reading

1. Guidelines for the diagnosis and management of multiple myeloma, 2014. British Committee for Standards in Haematology. www.bcshguidelines.com.

16

Q1 What investigations might you consider for a patient with AKI?

Initial bloods should be FBC, U&E (including bicarbonate), LFTs, calcium, phosphate and CRP. Baseline investigations should include a urine dip for blood and protein plus a renal ultrasound scan within 24 h if the cause of AKI is not immediately obvious. Other tests which may help but are not required in every case are CXR, ECG, blood gases, clotting screen, myeloma and vasculitis screens, as clinically indicated. Urine and blood should be sent for culture if infection is suspected. CT abdomen may be required when renal ultrasound shows no evidence of obstruction in circumstances in which obstruction seems likely while renal biopsy is the only certain way of confirming diagnoses of interstitial nephritis and systemic vasculitis.

Q2 Describe the principles of management of a patient with acute kidney injury.

Management should be determined by the cause, severity and any complications that may have developed. Most patients are dry, some will be shocked and for both of these groups of patients early fluid resuscitation is key. Fluid and everything else that needs to be done to treat AKI may conveniently be considered under the following headings:

Box 16.1 Key Issues to Consider in Management of AKI
- Reversible factors
- Specific therapies
- Organ failures
- Complications
- Bleeding risk
- Infection risk
- Nutritional
- Drugs

Q3 Discuss the management of reversible factors in AKI.

Essentially this means giving fluid if dry, stopping nephrotoxins, treating sepsis and relieving obstruction. The sicker the patient the more likely they are to require a urinary catheter in order to monitor urine output. Fluid management is so important that we devote a separate chapter to it. Guidelines recommend establishing a diuresis of over 30 ml/h though nephrologists much prefer 100 ml/h!

Q4 What specific therapies may be indicated in acute kidney injury?

Specific therapies target those with specific pathologies e.g. relief of obstruction if obstructed; steroids for interstitial nephritis;

steroids and cyclophosphamide for systemic vasculitis plus plasma exchange if the AKI is severe; plasma exchange with fresh frozen plasma for adult HUS-TTP. No specific treatment is required for ATN other than restoring renal perfusion, treating sepsis if present and stopping nephrotoxic drugs.

Q5   Discuss the role of frusemide, dopamine and inotropes in the management of patients with AKI.

- **Frusemide** 100 mg IV may increase urine volume but does not reduce the need for dialysis, shorten hospital stay or improve survival, so its use is not generally recommended.
- **Dopamine** 2 μg/kg/min is a renal vasodilator that may increase urine volume but, like frusemide, does not reduce the need for dialysis, shorten hospital stay or improve survival. It is no longer recommended.
- **Inotropes** do have a role to play in the management of patients with AKI. Noradrenaline starting at 0.1 μg/kg/min is effective in patients who are septic and hypotensive despite adequate fluid replacement. Dobutamine starting at 5 μg/kg/min is more appropriate in those with cardiogenic shock in order to increase cardiac output.

Q6   Which organ failures may occur in patients with AKI and how are they treated?

Patients with AKI may have either single organ or multi organ failure. In those with multi organ failure the organs systems commonly affected are renal, respiratory and circulation requiring renal replacement therapy, ventilation and inotropes respectively. In our unselected series of 396 consecutive patients with AKI requiring renal replacement therapy, 56 % had single organ AKI and 44 % required ventilation. Most of those ventilated also needed inotropic support.

Q7   What are the indications for renal replacement therapy in AKI?

These are essentially the same as the indications for dialysis in a patient with chronic kidney disease, as follows:

Box 16.2 Indications to Commence Dialysis in AKI

- **Symptomatic uraemia** – i.e. high level of blood urea with symptoms of anorexia, nausea and/or vomiting.
- **Pulmonary oedema** – patients with AKI and pulmonary oedema do not usually respond to intravenous frusemide.
- **Severe hyperkalaemia** – especially if serum potassium >6.5 mmol/l in an oliguric patient.
- **Severe acidosis** – especially if serum bicarbonate <10 mmol/l and patient is hypotensive.
- **Uraemic pericarditis** – a pericardial rub or effusion is a clear indication to start dialysis.

The decision to start RRT in AKI should be a clinical one based on the fluid, electrolyte and metabolic status of each patient, made before the development of significant complications or as early as possible thereafter. As a general rule the sicker the patient is then the lower the urea will be at the time of their first treatment. It is not uncommon to start dialysis in a patient whose urea is only 20 mmol/l if they have multi organ failure.

Q8   Does it matter whether renal replacement therapy is given by haemodialysis or haemofiltration?

The short answer to this question is no. Intensivists may favour haemofiltration because this is easier to do while nephrologists will probably prefer haemodialysis because this offers a wider range of treatment options including extended duration dialysis (EDD) and sustained low efficiency dialysis (SLED). A Cochrane Review failed to show a benefit of haemofiltration over haemodialysis when end points such as recovery of renal function and survival were compared. The principles of haemodialysis and haemofiltration are shown below (Fig. 16.1)

Fig. 16.1 Haemodialysis (*left*) uses diffusion to remove solutes from an area of high concentration (plasma) to an area of low concentration (dialysate) across a semipermeable membrane. Haemofiltration (*right*) uses convection to push water and solutes across a semipermeable membrane. Ultrapure replacement fluid is returned to the patient along with their filtered plasma

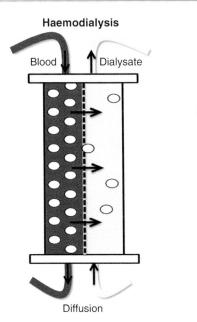

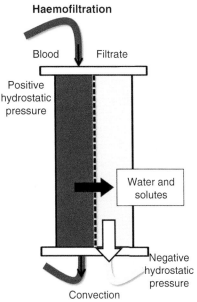

Q9   Give two life threatening complications of AKI

These are hyperkalaemia and pulmonary oedema. The management of hyperkalaemia is discussed in detail in a subsequent chapter. Pulmonary oedema in a patient with severe AKI is usually an indication for RRT, though in patients with lesser degrees of AKI it may be possible to establish a diuresis with intravenous diuretic.

Q10   Why are patients with AKI at greater risk of bleeding and what should be done about this?

Patients with AKI are more likely to bleed because their platelets are not as sticky, because they may require heparin to prevent their dialysis filters from clotting and because they are more prone to peptic ulceration. Because of this it is recommended that DVT prophylaxis, treatment of venous thromboembolism and acute coronary syndrome should be with half the normal recommended dose of low molecular weight heparin.

Q11   Why should you have a low threshold for considering infection in a patient with AKI?

Infection can be both cause and consequence of AKI. Sepsis as an important cause of pre-renal

AKI is discussed in an earlier chapter. Patients with AKI may become septic without developing a high fever which means a high index of suspicion is required. Essentially this means that if a patient with AKI looks unwell for no very obvious reason then you should consider blood culture, urine culture and chest x-ray.

Q12   What are the nutritional requirements of a patient with AKI and how may these be met?

Patients with severe AKI will lose their appetite while the AKI itself is usually catabolic. All patients with severe AKI should have nutritional review by a renal dietician who will usually recommend nutritional supplements and may also advise enteral (if the gut is working) feeding or parenteral nutrition (if it is not). The latest Renal Association guidelines recommend 20–35 kcal/kg/day and up to 1.7 g amino acids/kg/day if hypercatabolic and receiving continuous renal replacement therapies. Trace elements and water soluble vitamins may need to be supplemented.

Q13   Why is it important to review the drug kardex of patients with AKI?

Some drugs will be nephrotoxic while others will have side effects that become more troublesome in patients with AKI. Ten important neph-rotoxins are listed in the first of our chapters on AKI. Examples of drugs that may cause side effects because they cannot be excreted in patients with AKI include opiates, many antibiotics and low molecular weight heparin.

Q14 What is the likely outcome of AKI?

It used to be taught that patients with AKI either died with their renal failure, but not of it, or recovered renal function. Although most survivors of AKI have made at least a partial recovery of their renal function by the time of discharge from the hospital, it is now recognised that some will not. The literature also suggests that hospital mortality has remained around 50 % despite

recent advances in therapy although many now believe that our apparent failure to improve outcome in patients with AKI reflects the fact that older patients with more co-morbidity and more organ failure are being treated than before. In our own series of 396 consecutive patients, those who required ventilation had a significantly worse 90-day survival than those who did not whereas underlying CKD did not predict such an early adverse outcome. By 5 years, patients who had been ventilated during the acute illness were no longer at increased risk whereas the adverse effect of underlying CKD was statistically significant (Fig. 16.2). Underlying CKD was also a strong predictor of the need for RRT during follow-up.

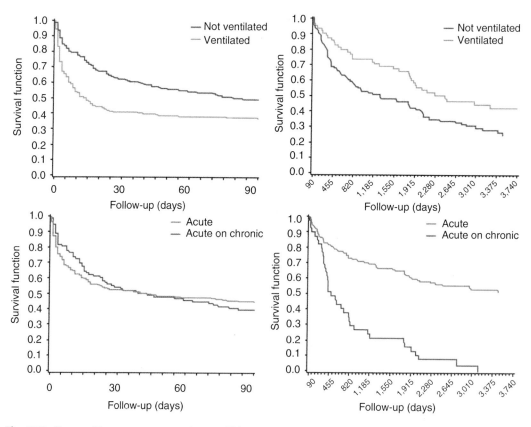

Fig. 16.2 Short and long term outcomes in acute kidney injury shown as survival against time. *Top two images*; ventilation carries a significantly higher chance of death in the short term which is no longer present at 5–10 years. *Bottom two images*; presence of underlying CKD confers no significant impact in the short term but reveals much

poorer outcomes in long term follow-up (Findlay M, et al. Chronic kidney disease rather than illness severity predicts medium- to long-term mortality and renal outcome after acute kidney injury. *Nephrol Dial Transplant*. 2014. First published online: 14 May 2014 by permission of Oxford University Press)

16.1 Objectives: Investigation, Management and Outcome of Acute Kidney Injury

After reading this chapter, you should be able to answer the following:

Q1 What investigations might you consider for a patient with AKI?

Q2 Describe the principles of management of a patient with acute kidney injury

Q3 Discuss the management of reversible factors in AKI.

Q4 What specific therapies may be indicated in acute kidney injury?

Q5 Discuss the role of frusemide, dopamine and inotropes in the management of patients with AKI.

Q6 Which organ failures may occur in patients with AKI and how are they treated?

Q7 What are the indications for renal replacement therapy in AKI?

Q8 Does it matter whether renal replacement therapy is given by haemodialysis or haemofiltration?

Q9 Give two life threatening complications of AKI

Q10 Why are patients with AKI at greater risk of bleeding and what should be done about this?

Q11 Why should there be a low threshold for considering infection in a patient with AKI?

Q12 What are the nutritional requirements of a patient with AKI and how may these be met?

Q13 Why is it important to review the drug kardex of patients with AKI?

Q14 What is the likely outcome of AKI?

Further Reading

1. Renal Association Clinical Practice Guideline for acute kidney injury, 2011. Available at www.renal.org/guidelines/modules/acute-kidney-injury.

Fluid Management

17

We have included a separate chapter on fluid management because most patients with acute kidney injury are dry requiring fluid replacement and many will be septic, requiring fluid resuscitation.

Q1 Describe the different body fluid compartments

Total body water makes up around 60 % of total body weight. This means that for a 75 kg person body water will be about 45 litres. Two third of this (30 litres) is intracellular and one third (15 litres) is extracellular. Two thirds of the extracellular fluid (approximately 10 litres) is interstitial and 1/3 (approximately 5 litres) is intravascular (plasma). The three body compartments are separated by membranes with different permeabilities: both are freely permeable to water but only capillary membranes are freely permeable to electrolytes (Fig. 17.1).

Q2 What is normal fluid intake and output?

Normal intake is around 2,000 ml/day and normal output 1,500 ml urine plus 500 ml insensible losses. Healthy individuals can of course cope with higher and lower intakes, principally by the effects of aldosterone and ADH on urine output. Medical students who feel they need to sip water from a plastic bottle on ward rounds in order to keep themselves adequately hydrated can be reassured!

Q3 Name three things that can go wrong with fluid balance?

There may be an imbalance between input and output, redistribution of fluid or an osmolar problem. Imbalance means either too much or too little fluid and is the easiest of the three to measure. Redistribution occurs as a result of leaky capillaries. This is driven by large plasma proteins especially albumin which is responsible for keeping fluid inside capillaries in health and which leaks

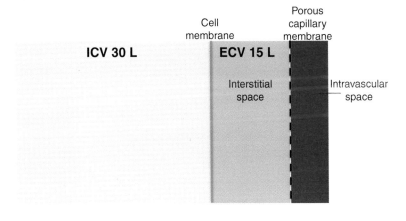

Fig. 17.1 Body fluid compartments. *ICV* intracellular volume, *ECV* extracellular volume

out into the tissues taking fluid with it when a patient becomes unwell. Osmolar problems across cell membranes including the blood brain barrier are driven by the concentration of small diffusible ions, mainly Na, K, glucose and urea. Together these ions exert a 'pressure' which causes water to move across cell membranes from weaker to stronger solutions until the concentration of solutes is equal on both sides. The classic example of this is cerebral oedema which occurs when water moves into the brain e.g. in acute hyponatraemia.

Q4 How might you decide whether a patient is dry, wet or euvolaemic?

A patient with vomiting, diarrhoea, excessive stoma losses or inadequate fluid intake is almost certainly going to be dry, but in the absence of such obvious clues assessment of fluid volume status is often trickier than it looks. No single sign is sufficiently sensitive and specific to confirm or exclude hypovolaemia and clinical assessment must be interpreted in context of history and relevant lab results. The signs shown in the box below have been taken from the Academy of Royal Colleges AKI Competency Framework. A postural rise in pulse and fall in blood pressure may be detected by sitting a patient up rather than asking them to stand, if too unwell to do so. Other clues to dryness include a urea:creatinine ratio >100:1 (normal range is 60–80:1). Urine/plasma osmolality greater than 1.1 and urine sodium <20 mmol/l also suggests dryness though these tests have little added value in most patients. CVP measurement does not have a role in the routine assessment of volume status.

Box 17.1 Assessment of Fluid Volume Status
1. Postural changes in pulse and blood pressure*
2. Dryness of axillae*
3. Moistness of mucous membranes
4. Skin turgor
5. Jugular venous pressure
6. Capillary refill time
7. Changes in body weight
8. Urine output and fluid balance chart
9. Peripheral or pulmonary oedema, pleural effusions, ascites

---

10. Physiological response to a fluid challenge*

*said to be the most useful signs of dryness

Q5 Is it possible to be intravascularly dry and yet oedematous at the same time?

Yes. Redistribution of fluid as a result of leaky capillaries in a septic patient is perhaps the commonest clinical scenario. Patients with massive leg oedema and/or ascites may well be dry intravascularly as indeed can occasional patients with pulmonary oedema (the classical scenario being right ventricular infarction). It is of course always more difficult to assess for dryness in a patient who is 'wet' and such patients are certainly more difficult to manage than those without oedema, simply because the underlying problem cannot usually be corrected by giving large volumes of intravenous fluid. The combination of cardiac and renal failure is often called cardiorenal failure, which we discuss in more detail in Chap. 12.

Q6 How might you calculate how much fluid to give?

The latest NICE guideline on IV Fluid replacement suggests that calculation of fluid requirements for any patient, including those with AKI, can conveniently be considered under three headings:

Resuscitation – to restore circulation to vital organs following loss of intravascular volume

Replacement – to treat any deficits or ongoing losses not needed urgently for resuscitation

Maintenance – any patient not drinking/unable to drink/having to fast for over 8–12 h should be started on IV maintenance fluid (Fig. 17.2)

Requirement for fluid =

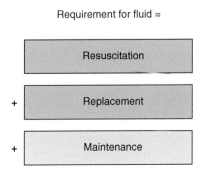

Fig. 17.2 Formula for calculating fluid requirements

Fig. 17.3 Distribution of fluids throughout body compartments

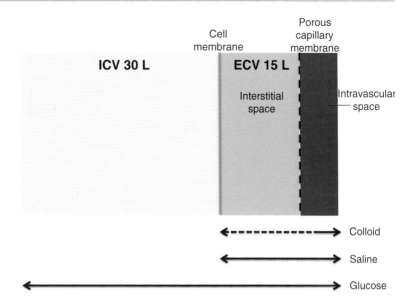

Q7 How much and which fluid for resuscitation?

Patients with significant co-morbidities and those taking cardiovascular drugs may become shocked with little fluid loss whereas young fit patients can compensate for much greater loss of intravascular volume. Start with a fluid bolus of 500 ml over 15 min and follow with further fast fluid up to 20 ml/kg if signs suggest still needs fluid resuscitation. Keep reassessing and have a low threshold for seeking expert help. The fluid can be crystalloid or colloid but not dextrose. Colloid is best at expanding intravascular space (1 litre gelaspan is equivalent to 2 litres saline) but is more expensive, carries a risk of anaphylaxis and hasn't been shown to improve outcome in resuscitation: because of this we tend to use crystalloid instead.

Q8 How much fluid for replacement?

Replacement fluid is required for patients who are dry but not shocked. Replacement fluid is for existing deficits and/or ongoing losses, both of which can be difficult to quantify: calculation of interstitial (capillary leak) losses is largely a matter of educated guesswork, fluid balance and daily weight charts are notoriously inaccurate, and insensible losses can increase significantly with exercise, fever and raised ambient temperature.

Q9 Which fluid for replacement?

Saline 0.9 % and Hartmann's are crystalloid replacement fluids. Both may be used to expand the intravascular space and both are more effective than dextrose for replacement because their sodium content restricts distribution to extracellular space. Hartmann's is the more physiological of the two. Dextrose loses the osmotic effect of glucose as it is rapidly metabolised and so moves into intracellular space (Fig. 17.3). Plasmalyte is more physiological than Hartmann's and may ultimately replace Hartmann's, though for the time being Hartmann's is crystalloid of choice for fluid replacement unless:

- Serum Na >145 mmol/l (could reduce osmolarity too quickly)
- Serum Cl <95 mmol/l (insufficient Cl)
- Serum K >6 mmol/l (because contains K)
- Head injury (risk of cerebral oedema because slightly hypo-osmolar)
- Hepatic failure (may be unable to convert lactate into bicarbonate)

Q10 Normal saline isn't normal. Discuss.

Saline 0.9 % is generally referred to as normal saline because it used to be thought that its salt concentration was similar to that of plasma. This is now known not to be the case. The main drawback of saline 0.9 % is that large volumes can load the extracellular fluid compartment with

Table 17.1 Composition of IV fluids

Fluid	Na (mmol/l)	K (mmol/l)	Chloride (mmol/l)	Osm (mosm/l)
Plasma	136–145	3.5–5.2	98–105	280–300
Saline 0.9 %	154	0	154	308
Hartmann's[a]	131	5	111	275
Plasmalyte[b]	140	5	98	294
Gelaspan[c]	151	4	103	284
Dextrose 5 %[d]	0	0	0	278

Other constituents are
[a]Lactate 29 mmol/l
[b]Acetate 27 mmol/l and gluconate 23 mmol/l
[c]Gelatin 40 g/l
[d]Dextrose 50 g/l

more sodium and chloride than is necessary. Five litres saline 0.9 % contains 1,540 mOsm of solute which sick patients may take up to 5 days to excrete. The retained chloride may reduce GFR and also cause a hyperchloraemic acidosis. The only clear indication for saline 0.9 % is vomiting with hypochloraemia. The composition of saline 0.9 % and other prescribed fluids is shown in Table 17.1

Q11   How much fluid for maintenance?
Maintenance daily fluid requirements for a healthy adult are:

> **Box 17.2 Maintenance Fluid Requirements for Healthy Adult**
> * Water 30 ml/kg
> * Sodium 1 mmol/kg
> * Potassium 1 mmol/kg
> * Calories 50–100 g/day of glucose to limit starvation ketosis

NICE recommend that we do not exceed 30 ml/kg/day and consider prescribing less maintenance fluid for patients who are obese, older, frail or have renal impairment or cardiac failure

Q12   Which fluid for maintenance?
The conventional approach is to give dextrose 5 % with saline 0.9 % and added K in ratio 3 dextrose: 1 saline. For a healthy 70 kg adult 3×500 ml dextrose and 1×500 ml saline 0.9 % given 6 hourly with 40 mmol added K per day

will give 2,000 ml fluid, 77 mmol Na, 40 mmol K and 300 cal. You could also consider 0.18 % saline in 4 % dextrose (dextrose-saline) with added K when prescribing for routine maintenance only. For a healthy 70 kg adult, 2,100 ml dextrose-saline (30 ml/kg) prescribed at 87 ml/h using 1 litre bags will supply all volume, Na, K and calorie needs for up to 3 days. Bear in mind that maintenance fluid is intended for short periods only and consider enteral feeding if the patient hasn't started eating and drinking by then.

Q13   When should you give IV fluid to a patient with acute kidney injury?
When the clinical history, signs and lab results suggest they might be dry (see Box 17.1). In every day clinical practice it is generally safe to assume an AKI patient is dry if there is no oedema, no elevation of the JVP, no dyspnoea, no basal crackles and normal SpO_2. It goes without saying that patients who appear shocked should receive IV fluid.

Q14   How much IV fluid should you give a patient with acute kidney injury?
Your aim should be to give as much fluid as required in order to restore renal perfusion, as quickly as possible. Shocked patients with AKI should receive 20 ml/kg crystalloid stat. For patients with AKI who are dry but not shocked we commonly give 1 litre in the first hour, then 1 litre over 2 h and 1 litre in the next 4 h i.e. 3 litres in the first 7 h. Junior doctors who prescribe 4 hourly bags as replacement fluid need to be aware that 4 hourly bags usually take 5 h to run on a general ward i.e. 100 ml/h. IV fluid

delivered at this rate is equivalent to taking more than 3 h to drink a can of coke.

Q15 What should you do if uncertain whether patient dry or not?

The correct course of action here is to give a fluid challenge of 250 ml saline 0.9 % or Hartmann's, squeezed in over 2–3 min followed by immediate assessment of clinical response. If the heart rate decreases and the blood pressure increases this suggests that the patient was in fact hypovolaemic and should lead to a further fluid challenge i.e. a fluid challenge is only a 'test dose' and is not enough in its own right to correct renal perfusion. More fluid must then be given. The renal target is a urine volume >30 ml/h, though if you want to make a nephrologist really happy you should ensure that your patient is passing more than 100 ml urine per hour!

Q16 What if the patient has a history of heart failure?

Patients with a history of heart failure are more likely to develop pulmonary oedema during or after a fluid challenge. A rising respiratory rate is the earliest sign, followed by increasing oxygen requirement then basal crackles. This is not a reason to withhold a fluid challenge, merely advice to be more cautious by infusing lower volumes of fluid less quickly than for patients without cardiac disease. Some patients with AKI also have evidence of cardiac failure at the time of presentation. This is known as cardiorenal failure, which makes everything much more complicated. We discuss a strategy for fluid management in cardiorenal failure in more detail in Chap. 12.

17.1   Objectives: Fluid Challenge

After reading this chapter, you should be able to answer the following:

Q1 Describe the different body fluid compartments

Q2 What is normal fluid intake and output?

Q3 Name three things that can go wrong with fluid balance?

Q4 How might you decide whether a patient is dry, wet or euvolaemic?

Q5 Is it possible to be intravascularly dry and oedematous at the same time?

Q6 How might you calculate how much fluid to give?

Q7 How much and which fluid for resuscitation?

Q8 How much fluid for replacement?

Q9 Which fluid for replacement?

Q10 Normal saline isn't normal. Discuss.

Q11 How much fluid for maintenance?

Q12 Which fluid for maintenance?

Q13 When should you give IV fluid to a patient with acute kidney injury?

Q14 How much IV fluid should you give a patient with acute kidney injury?

Q15 What should you do if uncertain whether patient dry or not?

Q16 What if the patient has a history of heart failure?

Further Reading

1. National Institute for Health and Care Excellence. Intravenous fluid therapy for adults in hospital. (Clinical guideline 174.) 2013. www.nice.org.uk/CG174.

Hyperkalaemia

Q1 How does your knowledge of potassium homeostasis help in the diagnosis and management of hyperkalaemia?

The diagram we used in Chap. 1 to describe potassium homeostasis can also be used to illustrate the pathophysiology of hyperkalaemia. Dietary potassium is of the order 50–100 mmol/day. Most of this is stored intracellularly. Excretion is predominantly renal. Acute and chronic kidney injury are important causes of hyperkalaemia as is the acidosis of acute illness. Figure 18.1 also suggests three ways in which potassium may be driven back into cells: by insulin, by beta agonists such as salbutamol and by correction of acidosis.

Q2 What is the normal range for serum potassium and at what point would you regard a patient as being hyperkalaemic?

The normal range is 3.5–5.4 mmol/l. The latest UK Renal Guidelines define hyperkalaemia as mild (serum K^+ 5.5–5.9 mmol/l), moderate (serum K^+ 6.0–6.4 mmol/l) or severe (serum $K^+ \geq 6.5$ mmol/l). Others use 7.0 mmol/l as the threshold for severe hyperkalaemia. It probably doesn't matter hugely whether 6.5 mmol/l or 7.0 mmol/l is taken as a cut point. What matters more is the rate at which serum potassium is rising and the likelihood it will rise further.

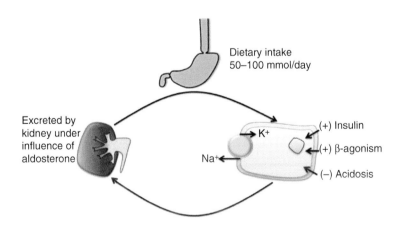

Fig. 18.1 Potassium homeostasis

Q3   Give the causes of hyperkalaemia.

The most important are acute and chronic renal failure. Many of the other causes begin with A as shown in Box 18.1. This list is not intended to be exhaustive. For a more complete list of all drugs associated with hyperkalaemia, see the Renal Association guideline.

Box 18.1 Causes of Hyperkalaemia

<u>A</u>cute and chronic kidney injury

<u>A</u>drenal failure

<u>A</u>cidosis

<u>A</u>rtefact (haemolysis)

<u>A</u>CE inhibitor

<u>A</u>ngiotensin receptor blocker

<u>A</u>ldosterone antagonist (spironolactone)

<u>A</u>nti-inflammatory drug (NSAID)

<u>A</u>ntibiotic (specifically trimethoprim)

Q4   What are the risks of hyperkalaemia?

Many medical students answer this question by saying 'arrhythmia'. This is not precise enough. The particular risk of hyperkalaemia is death by asystole or VF. Narrow complex tachycardia including atrial fibrillation, ventricular tachycardia and idioventricular rhythms have also been reported.

Q5   How does hyperkalaemia present clinically?

Sudden death is common as many patients will be completely asymptomatic until they present with asystole or VF. Others may complain of nausea, fatigue, muscle weakness or paraesthesia before developing such serious complications.

Q6   What are the ECG changes of hyperkalaemia?

Although the pattern of ECG changes can vary from patient to patient the following sequence is most commonly seen:

Box 18.2 Common Sequence of ECG Changes with Increasing Hyperkalaemia

1. Peaked T waves are an early sign
2. Loss of the P wave
3. Widening of the QRS complex
4. Bradycardia
5. Asystole

The ECG will usually be available before the serum biochemistry. You should suspect life threatening hyperkalaemia if an ECG shows bradycardia, broad complexes and no obvious P waves. The absence of P waves distinguishes life threatening hyperkalaemia from complete heart block (Fig. 18.2).

Q7   When should you treat hyperkalaemia?

The decision to treat should be based on the level of potassium, the likelihood it will rise further and the presence of ECG changes. In practice this means always treating when serum K $\geq$6.5 mmol/l and usually treating when serum K is 6.0–6.4 mmol/l (Fig. 18.3).

Q8   How would you treat hyperkalaemia in the acute setting?

The Renal Association suggest five key steps in the management of hyperkalaemia and that we should never walk away until all five have been addressed (Fig. 18.4).

We summarise the management of the first three of these steps in Fig. 18.5.

Q9   Discuss the use of intravenous calcium for hyperkalaemia in AKI.

- Protects heart but does not lower serum K.
- The recommended dose is 6.8 mmol which is achieved by giving calcium chloride 10 ml 10 % IV or calcium gluconate 30 ml 10 % IV

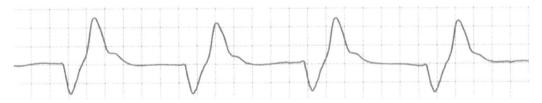

Fig. 18.2 ECG changes of hyperkalaemia (Note peaked T waves, absence of P waves, broad QRS and profound bradycardia)

Fig. 18.3 Factors influencing treatment choices in hyperkalaemia

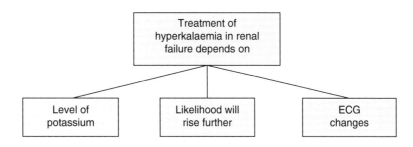

Fig. 18.4 Five key steps to address before you walk away (Reproduced with permission from Clinical Practice Guidelines. Treatment of acute hyperkalaemia in Adults. UK Renal Association, 2014)

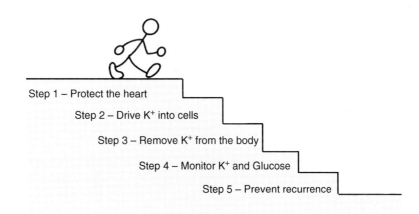

Fig. 18.5 Treatment principles in hyperkalaemia

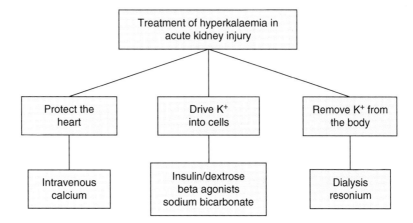

- Indicated if there are any ECG changes, repeating every 3–5 min until rate increases and QRS narrows.
- Onset of action is within minutes.
- May precipitate if given in the same line as bicarbonate.
- Calcium chloride is more likely to cause tissue necrosis if extravasates (Fig. 18.6) so better to use calcium gluconate if you cannot be sure of the vein.

Q10 Discuss the use of insulin dextrose for hyperkalaemia in AKI.
- The recommended ratio of insulin to dextrose is 10 units insulin: 25 g dextrose
- Until very recently, routine practice was to give 10 units soluble insulin with 50 ml 50 % dextrose IV over 15–30 min. Unfortunately, extravasation of such high concentrations of dextrose can lead to tissue necrosis (as can calcium, above). As a result

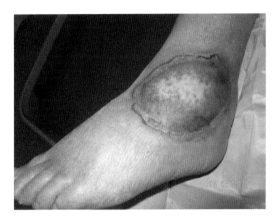

Fig. 18.6 Tissue necrosis caused by extravasation of intravenous calcium chloride

many units are now recommending adding 10 units soluble insulin to 250 ml 10 % dextrose and infusing this over 15–30 min.

- This will begin to take effect within 15 min and will lower serum potassium by 1–2 mmol/l for 1–2 h before gradually wearing off by 4–6 h.
- The Renal Association recommend monitoring blood glucose every 15 min for 1 h, every 30 min for the second hour then hourly for up to 6 h, because of the risk of hypoglycaemia
- Insulin may be given without dextrose in diabetic ketoacidosis at least until the BG is less than 14 mmol/l.

Q11   Discuss the use of salbutamol for hyperkalaemia in AKI.

- The recommended dose of salbutamol for hyperkalaemia is 10–20 mg by nebuliser or 500 μg IV over 10 min. Note that these doses are much higher than those used in asthma or COPD.
- This will begin to take effect at 30–60 min and will lower serum K by around 1 mmol/l for up to 2 h.
- Salbutamol may be ineffective as monotherapy in up to 40 % patients with hyperkalaemia and is best given in combination with insulin and dextrose.
- Most patients given salbutamol will have bradycardia initially because of their hyper-

kalaemia, though for those who are tachycardic the dose may need to be reduced.

Q12   Discuss the use of sodium bicarbonate for hyperkalaemia in AKI.

- The routine use of sodium bicarbonate for the management of acute hyperkalaemia is no longer recommended
- There may be a case for giving bicarbonate in combination with insulin, dextrose and salbutamol to AKI patients with hyperkalaemia if they are also profoundly acidotic
- Under these circumstances 500 ml of 1.26 % solution (75 mmol) over 60 min may lower serum K by an additional 0.5 mmol/l with onset of action 30–60 min, duration 3–4 h.

Q13   Discuss the use of calcium resonium for hyperkalaemia in AKI.

- This is a cation exchange resin which is not absorbed and which exchanges calcium for potassium across the bowel wall even if the patient is not eating.
- The usual dose is 15 G qds orally with water. Patients will become constipated after a few doses so add lactulose 10 ml tds and senna 2 tabs at night.
- Can give 30 g as an enema in methylcellulose solution if nil orally, repeating every 4–6 h if necessary. Colon must be irrigated to remove resin between doses.
- Onset of action after 4 h with peak effect at 24 h – therefore no place in emergency management, but may have a role in mild to moderate hyperkalaemia where control over a longer period of time may be acceptable and in circumstances where dialysis is delayed or inappropriate.

Q14   Discuss the use of dialysis for hyperkalaemia in AKI.

- Dialysis is the definitive treatment for hyperkalaemia as shown by the case history that follows (see below)
- Will lower serum K by 1 mmol/l in first hour and by further 1 mmol/l in next 2 h.

Case Report

AA 67 year old woman developed diarrhoea while taking enalapril and frusemide for hypertension. She was semiconscious when first seen with GCS 6/15, bradycardia 20 per minute and blood pressure 40/0 mmHg. Her ECG showed broad complexes with no P waves. Initially she was given dextrose and insulin and paced, but did not improve. By this time her initial bloods were available showing serum potassium 9.4 mmol/l, blood urea 42.6 mmol/l and serum creatinine 598 μmol/l. Thirty ml of 10 % calcium chloride led to a dramatic increase in heart rate and serum potassium fell to 4.4 mmol/l with emergency dialysis. The cause of this patient's hyperkalaemia was AKI precipitated by diarrhoea while taking an ACE inhibitor. Her ACE inhibitor was reintroduced on recovery and her potassium was 4.7 with urea 7.9 mmol/l and creatinine 86 μmol/l when last seen at the clinic.

McGuigan J et al. Life threatening hyperkalaemia with diarrhoea during ACE inhibition. *Emerg Med J.* 2005;22(2):154–155; with permission from BMJ Publishing Group Ltd

Q15 What would you recommend for a patient with AKI, serum K 6.4 mmol/l but no ECG changes?

- Calcium chloride not needed.
- Insulin/dextrose as above
- Unlikely to need salbutamol or bicarbonate.
- Consider calcium resonium unless likely to require dialysis immediately, otherwise start dialysis.

Q16 What would you recommend for a patient with AKI, serum K 6.4 mmol/l with ECG changes?

- Give calcium gluconate 10 % 30 ml IV repeated every 3–5 min until QRS complex has narrowed, to a maximum of 90 ml IV.
- Insulin/dextrose as above.

- Salbutamol 10–20 mg by nebuliser.
- Consider sodium bicarbonate 500 ml 1.26 % if acidotic.
- Consider emergency dialysis.

Q17 What should be done if hyperkalaemia is discovered during a cardiac arrest?

- Adrenaline 1 mg IV if not already given will help push potassium into the cells and out of the circulation, as adrenaline is a beta-agonist like salbutamol.
- Calcium chloride 10 ml 10 % IV.
- Insulin/dextrose as above
- Salbutamol 20 mg by nebuliser.
- Sodium bicarbonate 50 ml 8.4 % solution over 5 min.
- Consider emergency dialysis.

Q18 How does the treatment of hyperkalaemia in chronic renal failure differ?

Serum K of 6.4 mmol/l in a regular dialysis patient is likely to be less dangerous than the same level in an anuric catabolic acute. The former is usually a steady state whereas in the latter the potassium is only likely to rise further. Both patients should have an ECG looking for loss of P waves and broadening of QRS complex. If there are no ECG changes in the patient with CKD (steady state hyperkalaemia) then dietary advice and a review of dialysis prescription will often be sufficient up to serum K of 6.5 mmol/l.

Q19 What steps would you take to prevent recurrence of hyperkalaemia?

In the acute setting the key to successful prevention is to remember that driving potassium into cells is only a temporary measure, buying time before potassium can be eliminated from the body. If insulin dextrose is given but not followed by dialysis or resonium and it is not possible to establish a urine output, then hyperkalaemia is more than likely to recur.

The main measures for preventing recurrence thereafter are regular blood monitoring, careful drug prescribing and dietary advice. ACE inhibitors, ARBs, NSAIDs and K sparing diuretics should either be used cautiously or avoided altogether in patients with established renal disease or residual renal impairment following an episode of AKI, particularly if complicated by hyperkalemia. Potassium containing salt substitutes such as Lo-Salt should also be avoided.

Patients attending a renal clinic who have had an episode of hyperkalaemia should be assessed by a renal dietician who will advise to avoid or reduce intake of potassium rich foods such as coffee, chocolate, fruit and vegetables (see Chap. 29 and Appendix 9). Recurrent hyperkalaemia in a dialysis patient should prompt the same steps and advice but will also require reassessment of dialysis adequacy and dialysis prescription (see Chap. 37).

18.1   Objectives: Hyperkalaemia

After reading this chapter, you should be able to answer the following;

Q1   How does your knowledge of potassium homeostasis help in the diagnosis and management of hyperkalaemia?

Q2   Give the normal range for serum potassium and at what point would you regard a patient as being hyperkalaemic?

Q3   Give the causes of hyperkalaemia.

Q4   What are the risks of hyperkalaemia?

Q5   When should you treat hyperkalaemia?

Q6   How does hyperkalaemia present clinically?

Q7   What are the ECG changes of hyperkalaemia?

Q8   How would you treat hyperkalaemia in the acute setting?

Q9   Discuss the use of intravenous calcium for hyperkalaemia in AKI.

Q10   Discuss the use of insulin dextrose for hyperkalaemia in AKI.

Q11   Discuss the use of salbutamol for hyperkalaemia in AKI.

Q12   Discuss the use of sodium bicarbonate for hyperkalaemia in AKI.

Q13   Discuss the use of calcium resonium for hyperkalaemia in AKI.

Q14   Discuss the use of dialysis for hyperkalaemia in AKI.

Q15   What would you recommend for a patient with AKI, serum K 6.4 mmol/l but no ECG changes?

Q16   What would you recommend for a patient with AKI, serum K 6.4 mmol/l with ECG changes?

Q17   What should be done if hyperkalaemia is discovered during a cardiac arrest?

Q18   How does the treatment of hyperkalaemia in chronic renal failure differ?

Q19   What steps would you take to prevent recurrence of hyperkalaemia?

Further Reading

1. Alfonzo A et al. Clinical Practice Guidelines. Treatment of acute hyperkaleaemia in adults. UK Renal Association, 2014. www.renal.org/guidelines/modules/treatment-of-acute-hyperkalaemia-in-adults.

Rapidly Progressive Glomerulonephritis

19

Q1 What do you understand by the term Rapidly Progressive Glomerulonephritis (RPGN)?

RPGN (also known as crescentic nephritis) is the most aggressive form of glomerulonephritis. It is characterised by sub-acute renal failure i.e. renal failure that develops over a matter of weeks rather than hours to days (acute kidney injury) or months to years (chronic kidney disease). It is important to recognise that if not suspected, diagnosed and treated as a matter of urgency then the renal failure is likely to be irrecoverable with patients becoming dialysis dependent permanently.

Q2 What are the causes of RPGN?

The most important causes are the ANCA positive systemic vasculitides; granulomatous polyarteritis (GPA) – previously "Wegener's Granulomatosis"- and microscopic polyarteritis (MPA). Anti-GBM disease, diffuse lupus nephritis and some forms of primary glomerulonephritis especially IgA nephropathy, may also present with rapidly progressive nephritis.

Box 19.1 Specific Causes of RPGN
- Granulomatous Polyarteritis (Wegener's)
- Microscopic Polyarteritis
- Anti-GBM disease
- Diffuse lupus nephritis
- Primary GN especially IgA nephropathy

Q3 When should you suspect RPGN?

When a patient presents with unexplained kidney injury and something else. It may be helpful to think of RPGN as 'Renal failure plus' in much the same way we think of 'Parkinson's plus' and 'Rheumatoid plus' syndromes. The most common 'plus' is the lung i.e. patient presents with a Pulmonary Renal Syndrome. Other organs/tissues that may be involved are the skin (vasculitic rash) and the nervous system (mononeuritis multiplex). The different types of other system involvement in patients with RPGN are summarised in Box 19.2.

Box 19.2 Presentation of RPGN
- Systemic e.g. fever, night sweats, weight loss, malaise (All)
- ENT involvement with sinusitis and otitis media (GPA) – saddle nose
- Dyspnoea, cough, haemoptysis (GPA, MPA, anti-GBM)
- Photosensitivity, arthralgia, skin rash (SLE)

Q4 What should you do if you suspect RPGN?

Confirming the diagnosis is essential to allowing timely management to preserve renal function. Patients will usually require:

1. An urgent vasculitis screen and
2. An urgent renal biopsy

M. Findlay, C. Isles, *Clinical Companion in Nephrology*,
DOI 10.1007/978-3-319-14868-7_19, © Springer International Publishing Switzerland 2015

Fig. 19.1 Classification of RPGN based on serum immunology testing

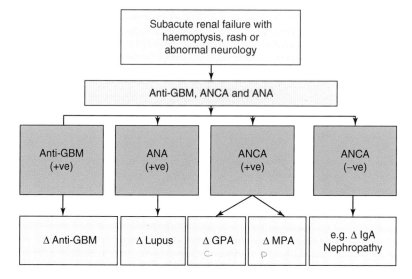

Q5 What is meant by an urgent vasculitis screen?

Patients with suspected RPGN should have a clotted blood sample sent urgently to Immunology for ANCA screen, ANA and anti-GBM antibodies. ANCA stands for anti-neutrophil cytoplasmic antibodies. Two specificities are recognised. Patients with GPA have high titres of anti-proteinase 3 (anti-PR3) antibody while those with MPA have high titres of anti-myeloperoxidase (anti-MPO) antibodies. These serological tests help distinguish five causes of RPGN as shown in Fig. 19.1:

Q6 What is the renal biopsy likely to show?

In patients with GPA, MPA and anti-GBM disease there will be a focal segmental necrotising glomerulonephritis with crescents, – hence "crescentic nephritis". Crescents are a non-specific response to severe inflammation of epithelial cells in the glomerulus resulting in a mixed cellular/fibrotic casing which can engulf the glomerulus. This give a half-moon (crescent) appearance on histological cross-section (Fig. 19.2). Immunofluorescence in GPA and MPA shows minimal deposition of immunoglobulins or complement, hence the term 'pauci-immune' glomerulonephritis, whereas immunofluorescence in anti-GBM disease reveals linear staining for IgG.

Q7 How would you manage a patient with GPA or MPA?

Briefly, when a patient presents with GPA or MPA and is found to have RGPN then he or she will likely receive:

Box 19.3 Acute Management of Vasculitis
1. High dose steroids (IV methyprediso-lone or oral prednisolone)
2. IV pulsed cyclophosphamide, the dose of which is determined by their age, serum creatinine and white cell count.
3. Seven plasma exchanges over the course of 2 weeks if baseline SC >500 µmol/l or pulmonary haemorrhage is present.

Because cyclophosphamide is a toxic drug (marrow suppression, infertility and haemorrhagic cystitis) guidelines advise a switch to azathioprine 1–2 mg/kg once remission has been achieved. More details on management of ANCA associated vasculitis are given in Appendix 7.

Q8 What do you know about anti-GBM disease?

Patients with anti-GBM disease present as rapidly progressively renal failure +/− haemoptysis. When haemoptysis is present this is known as Goodpasture's syndrome. The cause is an auto-antibody directed at the glomerular basement membrane, which also has activity against the pulmonary basement membrane. The diagnosis is made by finding anti-GBM antibodies in the blood stream with focal segmental necrotising GN, extensive crescents and linear deposition of IgG on the renal biopsy. Treatment is with high dose steroids

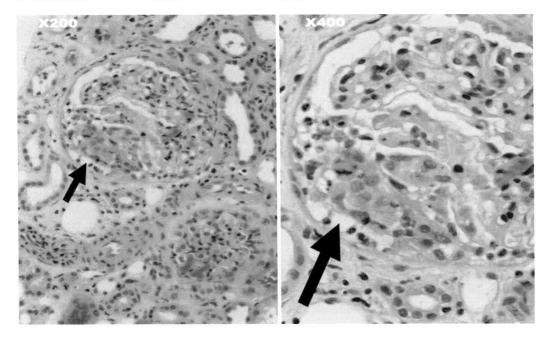

Fig. 19.2 Renal biopsy shows focal, segmental necrotising GN with early crescent at 7–9 o'clock (*arrowed*), magnified on the right

and IV pulse cyclophosphamide with plasma exchange until their anti-GBM antibody is no longer detectable.

Q9   What do you know about lupus nephritis?

SLE is a chronic inflammatory multisystem disease of unknown aetiology. It occurs most commonly in young women. Most patients will have an asymmetrical non deforming polyarthropathy with a butterfly rash on their face. Renal involvement occurs in up to 50 % of patients with SLE and may vary from mild (asymptomatic urinary abnormalities only) to severe (diffuse proliferative glomerulonephritis). The diagnosis of diffuse proliferative GN in lupus is made by serology and renal biopsy. First line treatment of diffuse proliferative lupus nephritis should be with high dose oral prednisolone and mycophenolate (see Chap. 36).

Q10   What is the outcome of RPGN?

It is difficult to give a hard and fast answer as this will depend on the age of the patient, the severity of their renal disease and the presence or absence of extra renal manifestations. In a recently published study of patients with GPA and MPA whose serum creatinine was greater

than 500 μmol/l initially, all of whom received oral cyclophosphamide and oral prednisolone, the proportion remaining dialysis dependent at 1 year was 20 % with plasma exchange and 40 % with intravenous methylprednisolone. One year survival was 75 % in each group.

Q11   What should you do if a patient with ANCA positive vasculitis relapses?

Relapse is usually defined as the occurrence of increased disease activity after a period of partial or complete remission. Relapses can be treated with steroids and cyclophosphamide and have a similar response rate as the initial disease. A difficulty may arise though if a patient has already received, or is likely to receive, 36 g cyclophosphamide as cumulative doses higher than this have been associated with a risk of malignancy. In these circumstances the latest guidelines suggest treating with a rituximab-based regimen. Rituximab is a monoclonal antibody against the protein CD20, which is found on the surface of B cells. Although the long-term safety of rituximab remains uncertain, its efficacy in relapse may provide an opportunity to minimize cumulative dosage and avoid the potential long-term toxicity of cyclophosphamide.

19.1   Objectives: Rapidly Progressive Glomerulonephritis

After reading this chapter, you should be able to answer the following:

Q1   What do you understand by the term Rapidly Progressive Glomerulonephritis (RPGN)?

Q2   What are the causes of RPGN?

Q3   When might you suspect RPGN?

Q4   What should you do if you suspect RPGN?

Q5   What is meant by an urgent vasculitis screen?

Q6   What is the renal biopsy likely to show?

Q7   How would you manage a patient with GPA or MPA?

Q8   What do you know about anti-GBM disease?

Q9   What do you know about lupus nephritis?

Q10   What is the outcome of RPGN?

Q11   What should you do if a patient with ANCA positive vasculitis relapses?

Further Reading

1. Jayne D, et al. Randomized trial of plasma exchange or high-dosage methylprednisolone as adjunctive therapy for severe renal vasculitis. J Am Soc Nephrol. 2007;18:2180–8.
2. Kidney Disease: Improving Global Outcomes (KDIGO) Glomerulonephritis Work Group. KDIGO Clinical Practice Guideline for Glomerulonephritis. Kidney Inter Suppl. 2012;2:139–274.

Q1 What is meant by the term chronic kidney disease?

A good working definition is an irreversible deterioration in renal function that develops over a period of months to years. This distinguishes chronic kidney disease from acute kidney injury which is best thought of as a deterioration in renal function, sometimes reversible and sometimes not, that develops over a period of hours to days. The current official definition of CKD includes all people with markers of kidney damage and those with GFR of less than 60 ml/min on at least 2 occasions separated by a period of at least 90 days. Markers of kidney damage are ACR more than 3 mg/mmol, urine sediment abnormalities, electrolyte and other abnormalities due to tubular disorders, abnormalities detected by histology, structural abnormalities detected by imaging and a history of kidney transplantation.

Q2 How common is chronic kidney disease?

The prevalence of CKD rises sharply with age and the frequency with which it is recognised has increased, some would argue artefactually, as a result of the widespread use of eGFR. For more details on how CKD is classified using the GFR see Chap. 2. Many elderly people are now classified as having CKD3 with eGFR 30–59 ml/min simply because of the formula used to calculate eGFR. Few of us would consider a person of 85 years of age with serum creatinine 120 umol/l to have chronic kidney disease any more than we would suggest that an elderly man or woman who had become slightly more breathless on exertion necessarily had chronic lung disease. Nephrons – like alveoli – have a tendency to wither with age. By complete contrast a serum creatinine of 120 umol/l in a teenager ought to set alarm bells ringing. These qualifications aside, the prevalence of CKD3 in the general population as determined by eGFR is around 5 % and that of CKD 4 and 5 around 0.2 % and 0.1 % respectively.

Q3 What are the symptoms of chronic kidney disease?

Many patients with chronic kidney disease are asymptomatic which means that their renal failure is only picked up when they have blood tests for something else. For patients who do have symptoms, many are non-specific, including nocturia, tiredness, and breathlessness. Anorexia and nausea indicate that dialysis may shortly be required in a patient whose renal failure is progressing, particularly if associated with weight loss. Generalised itch, often with scratch marks, and restless legs are more specific for chronic kidney disease than nocturia, tiredness and breathlessness, though they are not always present. Late symptoms, which one would hopes never to see, include hiccups, muscular twitching, fits, drowsiness and coma. The term 'uraemia' is usually taken to mean a high level of urea (often greater than 30 mmol/l) with loss of appetite, nausea or vomiting.

M. Findlay, C. Isles, *Clinical Companion in Nephrology*,
DOI 10.1007/978-3-319-14868-7_20, © Springer International Publishing Switzerland 2015

Box 20.1 Five symptoms that suggest progressive renal failure
1. Loss of appetite Anorexia
2. Nausea
3. Breathlessness
4. Generalised itch ⎤
5. Restless legs   ⎦ end stage

Q4   What are the signs of chronic kidney disease?

There aren't very many in the early stages of CKD. Oedema raises possibility of nephrotic syndrome but has numerous other causes. Palpable kidneys suggest autosomal dominant polycystic kidneys (ADPKD) but inability to feel one or both kidneys does not exclude this diagnosis. Increased bladder dullness is a useful and underrated sign in a patient with bladder neck obstruction. Patients with advanced CKD may be pale due to anaemia, pigmented due to uraemia and have scratch marks as a result of their pruritus. A pericardial friction rub means that it is time to start dialysis.

Box 20.2 Five signs that may be present in CKD
1. Oedema
2. Palpable kidneys (ADPKD)
3. Increased bladder dullness
4. Skin changes – pallor, pigmentation, scratch marks
5. Pericardial friction rub

Q5   What are the common causes of chronic kidney disease?

The pie chart shows the distribution of causes of all 533 patients who started renal replacement therapy in Scotland in 1999. Diabetes, glomerulonephritis and hypertensive renal diseases including renovascular disease were the three most frequently identified causes. Scottish Renal Registry data show that the causes of CKD

requiring dialysis today are very similar to those of 1999. Diabetes accounts for up to 40 % of the causes of kidney failure in patients on dialysis in some parts of the world. Glomerulonephritis is a term used to describe a number of disorders, most of them immunologically mediated, that primarily affect the glomeruli leading to chronic renal failure. The hallmark of glomerular disease is proteinuria. When hypertension causes kidney failure this is usually because of narrowing of the small blood vessels within the kidney, so called hypertensive nephrosclerosis. Renovascular disease and malignant hypertension are two other ways in which patients with hypertension may develop chronic renal failure (Fig. 20.1).

Tubulointerstitial diseases including chronic pyelonephritis, interstitial nephritis and analgesic nephropathy accounted for 12 % and polycystic kidneys for 8 % of the causes in the Scottish study. A heterogeneous group of causes including obstructive uropathy, myeloma, and SLE accounted for the remaining 14 % of causes. Note that in 24 % the cause of CKD could not be determined. Typically these were elderly patients

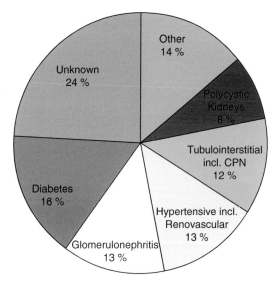

Fig. 20.1 Causes of chronic kidney disease (Metcalfe W et al. Equity of renal replacement therapy utilization: a prospective population-based study. *QJM: An International Journal of Medicine*. 1999;92;637–42, by permission of Oxford University Press)

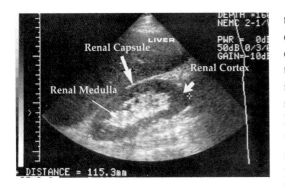

Fig. 20.2   Normal renal ultrasound appearance

with small kidneys on ultrasound precluding biopsy.

Q6   What investigations are most helpful in determining the cause of a patient's chronic kidney disease?

Without doubt the two most useful investigations are renal ultrasound together with urinalysis for blood and protein and quantification of proteinuria by ACR or PCR. Renal biopsy may be indicated in a proteinuric/haematuric patient with normal sized kidneys on ultrasound in order to establish a diagnosis of glomerulonephritis, interstitial nephritis or vasculitis. Serum immunology is not necessary in every case but complement, ANCA, ANA and anti-GBM, and occasionally cryoglobulins can be diagnostic when clinically indicated. Myeloma screen should be considered in the older patient particularly if anaemic, hypercalcaemic or has bone pain (see Chap. 15).

Box 20.3 Five useful investigations in CKD
1. Renal ultrasound
2. Urinalysis with urine ACR/PCR
3. Renal biopsy
4. Serum immunology.
5. Myeloma screen in the elderly.

If you know the patient's BP, blood glucose, renal ultrasound and urine ACR/PCR then it is possible to diagnose the likely cause of their CKD in most cases. Patients with diabetes have usually had the disease for several years before they develop proteinuria and renal failure. Glomerulonephritis should be suspected in a patient with small smooth kidneys, hypertension and proteinuria. A long history of hypertension without much proteinuria suggests that hypertensive nephrosclerosis may be the cause. The diagnosis of chronic pyelonephritis and polycystic kidneys is made by the characteristic appearances that are seen on renal ultrasound. Other diagnoses that can be confirmed or suggested by renal ultrasound are described in Q7.

Q7   What is the normal size of a kidney by renal ultrasound?

Normal renal length is 10–12 cm. The radiologists call this the bipolar diameter. Patients with bipolar diameter 9–10 cm have borderline small kidneys. Kidneys that are less than 9 cm in bipolar diameter are unequivocally small. There may well be a variation in renal size comparing right with left. Up to 1.5 cm difference in renal size can be within normal limits but more than 1.5 cm difference is abnormal (Fig. 20.2).

Q8   Discuss how renal ultrasound may help in the diagnosis of patients with chronic kidney disease.

This is all about pattern recognition. The following specific patterns of abnormality on ultrasound may either make or suggest a diagnosis:

The inequality of renal size in bilateral renovascular disease usually occurs because one renal artery occludes and the kidney shrinks as a result of the occlusion while the other kidney merely has a narrowed renal artery and a renal size that may still be normal. Patients with chronic kidney disease may also have normal sized kidneys of equal size with smooth outlines. From a practical point of view this is important as these are the kidneys which are safe to biopsy

Box 20.4 Five ways in which renal ultrasound may help

- Dilation of the pelvi-calyceal systems: Δ Obstructive Uropathy
- Both kidneys large & replaced by cysts of varying sizes: Δ Polycystic kidneys.
- Small smooth kidneys with heavy proteinuria: Δ Glomerulonephritis.
- Small scarred kidneys: Δ Chronic pyelonephritis.
- Unequal size: Δ Bilateral Reno-vascular Disease

Q9   Describe in broad terms the management of a patient with chronic kidney disease.

Management of CKD may conveniently be considered under the five headings in Box 20.5. Prevention of CKD progression, vascular disease and CKD complications are discussed here, while specific treatments, dialysis preparation and conservative care are covered in other chapter.

Box 20.5 Five key principles of management

1. Prevention of CKD progression
2. Prevention of vascular disease
3. Prevention and treatment of CKD complications
4. Specific measures for certain causes e.g. treatment of vasculitis and myeloma
5. Preparation for dialysis or conservative care

Q10   What are the risk factors for CKD progression?

The risk factors with which nephrologists are most familiar are hypertension and proteinuria. NICE have recently drawn our attention to others which include cardiovascular disease, acute kidney injury diabetes, smoking, African, African-Caribbean or Asian family origin, chronic use of NSAIDs and untreated urinary outflow tract obstruction.

Q11   How may CKD progression be prevented?

It is rare to completely halt or reverse CKD progression in a patient whose renal function has begun to deteriorate, but it is often possible to slow the rate at which renal function declines by controlling SBP to 120–140 mmHg and by the use of drugs that block the RAS in patients who have significant proteinuria (urine PCR >50 mg/mmol). Chronic use of NSAIDs should be avoided if at all possible and untreated urinary outflow tract obstruction should be considered, particularly in elderly men.

Q12   How may vascular disease be prevented?

Prevention of vascular disease is important because most patients with CKD will die of vascular disease and not of renal failure. All patients should receive lifestyle advice on diet, exercise and smoking. The latest NICE guideline suggests offering antiplatelet drugs to people with CKD for the secondary prevention of cardiovascular disease, while being aware of the increased risk of bleeding. The use of statins is more controversial. Both NICE and KDIGO recommend them for predialysis patients with CKD 3–5 though our interpretation of the literature is slightly different: namely that they are probably beneficial in CKD3 and possibly beneficial in CKD4. We are not convinced of their efficacy in CKD5, possibly because of the high incidence of LVH and arterial calcification in this patient group and so we tend to limit their use to predialysis CKD5 patients who have had a definite myocardial infarction and to those who are being considered for transplant.

Q13   How may the complications of CKD be prevented and treated?

Five important complications of CKD are anaemia, bone disease, hyperkalaemia, acidosis and malnutrition. The management of anaemia, bone disease and hyperkalaemia are discussed elsewhere. Declining renal function is associated with metabolic acidosis which in turn may exacerbate bone disease and increase catabolism. Most nephrologists will consider sodium bicarbonate 500 mg bd up to 1 g tds in order to maintain serum bicarbonate >20 mmol/l in patients with CKD4 and 5 while bearing in mind that this may cause or worsen oedema and hypertension. All patients with progressive CKD should be referred to a renal dietician for advice on protein, calorie, potassium and phosphate intake. Malnutrition is common and difficult to correct.

Box 20.6 Five complications of CKD
1. Anaemia
2. Bone disease
3. Hyperkalaemia
4. Acidosis
5. Malnutrition

Q14   How often should patients with CKD be reviewed?

The answer must be that it depends on the rate at which their renal function is declining. A good rule of thumb is that patients with CKD3 be reviewed every 6 months, CKD4 every 3 months and CKD5 every 6 weeks. Patients with CKD4/5 whose renal function is declining rapidly e.g. diabetic nephropathy with nephrotic range proteinuria may need to be seen more frequently than this in the run up to dialysis. Once you know, as a result of repeated measurements, that a patient's renal function is stable or only declining slowly then it is safe to extend the interval between reviews to annual for CKD3, every 6 months for CKD4 and every 3 months for CKD5.

20.1   Objectives: Chronic Kidney Disease

After reading this chapter, you should be able to answer the following:

Q1   What is meant by the term chronic kidney disease?

Q2   How common is chronic kidney disease?

Q3   What are the symptoms of chronic kidney disease?

Q4   What are the signs of chronic kidney disease?

Q5   What are the common causes of chronic kidney disease requiring dialysis?

Q6   What investigations are most helpful in determining the cause of a patient's chronic kidney disease?

Q7   What is the normal size of a kidney by renal ultrasound?

Q8   Discuss how renal ultrasound may help in the diagnosis of patients with chronic kidney disease.

Q9   Describe in broad terms the management of a patient with chronic kidney disease.

Q10   What are the risk factors for CKD progression?

Q11   How may CKD progression be prevented?

Q12   How may vascular disease be prevented?

Q13   How may the complications of CKD be treated and prevented?

Q14   How often should patients with CKD be reviewed?

Further Reading

1. Kidney Disease: Improving Global Outcomes (KDIGO) CKD Work Group. KDIGO 2012 Clinical Practice Guideline for the Evaluation and Management of Chronic Kidney Disease. Kidney Inter. Suppl. 2013;3:1–150.

2. National Institute for Health and Care Excellence. Chronic Kidney Disease: early identification and management of chronic kidney disease in primary and secondary care. CG182. London: National Institute for Health and Care Excellence; 2014.

3. Primary Renal Diagnosis of Patients starting Renal Replacement Therapy. Scottish Renal Registry Report 2013 with demographic data to 2013 and audit data to 2014. NHS National Services Scotland/Crown copyright 2013.

Glomerular Disease

Q1 What does the term glomerular disease mean?

Glomerular disease is a general term for a group of disorders affecting both kidneys in which there is usually, but not always, immunologically mediated injury to glomeruli, with renal interstitial damage a regular accompaniment. The clinical hallmark of glomerular disease is proteinuria.

Q2 Describe the pathophysiology of glomerular disease

The immunological insult is either by antigen antibody complexes deposited or formed on the glomerular basement membrane (GBM) or by antibodies directed towards the GBM. Antigen antibody complex deposition is thought to be the more common of the two mechanisms. The term 'glomerulonephritis' is often used to describe this group of disorders even if not all of them are due to inflammation.

Q3 How might you classify glomerular disease?

This is an area that medical students and junior doctors often find confusing. Glomerular disease can be classified by presentation, by cause and by pathology. The difficulty is that a particular presentation may have more than one cause and more than pathology. We have adopted a workable but simplified approach here.

Q4 How does glomerulonephritis present?

The glomerulus has a limited number of ways of responding to a variety of different stimuli. The following five clinical presentations of glomerular disease are recognised:

> **Box 21.1 Five presentations of glomerular disease**
> 1. Asymptomatic urinary abnormality i.e. proteinuria, haematuria or both
> 2. Acute nephritis
> 3. Nephrotic syndrome
> 4. Rapidly progressive renal failure
> 5. Chronic kidney disease

Q5 What is meant by asymptomatic urinary abnormalities?

The term describes patients whose only presenting features are asymptomatic proteinuria (i.e. not associated with oedema) or haematuria (which may be visible or non visible) or both. The detection and measurement of proteinuria and haematuria have been described in an earlier chapter

Q6 What do you understand by the term acute nephritis?

This is the name given to a syndrome that is no longer very common but usually occurs 10–14 days after an infection, classically a streptococcal sore throat. The features of acute nephritis are malaise, oliguria, hypertension, proteinuria (but not usually nephrotic range), haematuria (urine is often described as 'smoky' or 'coke coloured'), mild oedema and impaired renal function. Acute nephritis usually settles rapidly, although proteinuria and microscopic haematuria may persist for years. In a small proportion of patients the disease may become chronic, leading to renal failure.

Q7   What do you understand by the term nephrotic syndrome?

Nephrotic syndrome, which is more common in children than in adults, is characterised by the five features shown in Box 21.2. The cutpoints for proteinuria and hypoalbuminaemia required for diagnosis vary slightly depending on the textbook or guideline you happen to be reading – we have chosen urine PCR 350 mg/mmol and serum albumin 35 g/l because they are easy to remember.

Box 21.2 Five features of nephrotic syndrome
1. **Oedema**
2. **Proteinuria** with urine PCR >350 mg/mmol (equivalent to proteinuria >3.5 g/day).
3. **Hypoalbuminaemia** <35 g/l.
4. **Prothrombotic tendency.**
5. **Hyperlipidaemia.**

Patients with nephrotic syndrome can present with venous thrombo-embolism which occurs because their urinary protein loss includes fibrinolytic factors e.g. anti-thrombin III (see case history). They may also be hyperlipidaemic because their livers produce more lipoproteins as part of a generalised increase in protein synthesis to make up for the loss of protein in the urine.

Case Report

A 68 year old man presented with a swollen left leg and pleuritic chest pain. Ultrasononography confirmed a recent thrombus in the superficial femoral vein. He had dipstick urine of ++++ protein and a serum albumin of 24 g/l, both of which were overlooked at the time. Renal function was normal. The patient represented 2 months later with swelling of both legs while on warfarin with an INR of 1.3. Doppler showed a resolving DVT in the left superficial femoral vein but no DVT in the right leg. Urinalysis was not carried out on this occasion and a low serum albumin of 20 g/l was again overlooked. Three weeks later the general practitioner referred the patient for a third time as both legs were by now swollen to the upper thigh. A degree of redness led to a diagnosis of cellulitis and treatment with benzylpenicillin and flucloxacillin. Once again urinalysis was not performed and the serum albumin of 22 g/l was ignored. After discharge his GP noted heavy proteinuria and referred the patient directly to the Renal Unit where urine protein was quantified at 12.3 g/24 h and a diagnosis of nephrotic syndrome was confirmed. Renal biopsy showed that this was caused by membranous nephropathy.

Ambler B et al. Nephrotic syndrome presenting as deep vein thrombosis or pulmonary embolism. *Emergency Med J.* 2008;25:241–42; with permission from BMJ Publishing Group Ltd.

Q8   What do you understand by the term rapidly progressive renal failure?

This is an uncommon but extremely important presentation of glomerular disease. Rapidly progressive renal failure, sometimes known as sub-acute renal failure, is the usual clinical presentation of patients with granulomatous polyarteritis (previously Wegener's granulomatosis), microscopic polyarteritis, Goodpasture's syndrome and lupus nephritis. Early renal biopsy is essential as prompt immunosuppressive therapy may prevent permanent loss of renal function. Biopsy usually shows a focal and segmental necrotising glomerulonephritis with crescents (so called crescentic nephritis). This aggressive form of GN is discussed under renal emergencies.

Q9 Some patients with glomerular disease simply present with chronic renal failure. How would you make a diagnosis?

Patients who present with chronic renal failure and are found to have hypertension, heavy proteinuria and small smooth kidneys on ultrasound are generally assumed to have chronic glomerulonephritis. Renal biopsy is technically difficult in such patients, is more likely to be complicated by bleeding and often yields glomeruli in which the disease process is too far advanced to make a histological diagnosis. A diagnosis of probable rather than definite chronic GN is made therefore.

Box 21.3 Five causes of glomerular disease
1. **Idiopathic** – most cases of minimal change nephropathy, membranous nephropathy and FSGS
2. **Infective causes** e.g. post streptococcal, SBE, hepatitis B, hepatitis C
3. **Drugs** e.g. NSAIDs, previously gold and penicillamine
4. **Diabetes & other multi-system disorders** – a variety of diseases including diabetes, amyloid, SLE, Goodpasture's syndrome, granulomatous polyarteritis (GPA) & microscopic polyarteritis (MPA) may cause glomerular disease. The most important of these is diabetic nephropathy, the hallmark of which is proteinuria which will develop in up to 40 % of diabetics after 15–20 years.

5. **Malignancy** – myeloma can cause heavy proteinuria and may present with nephrotic syndrome. Some carcinomas e.g. bronchial carcinoma may be associated with membranous nephropathy and occasionally lymphoma may be associated with minimal change nephropathy.

Q10 What are the causes of glomerular disease?

Most cases of glomerular disease are idiopathic i.e. no known cause. Causes of glomerular disease can be considered under the following five headings:

Q11 Describe the histological features of glomerular disease.

This is a challenging area of nephrology. Biopsies that contain less than 10 glomeruli are difficult to interpret, particularly if the lesion happens to be focal (affecting only some glomeruli) or segmental (affecting only part of each glomerulus). A histological diagnosis is usually established by examining the appearances on light microscopy, immunofluorescence and electron microscopy and even then it is not always possible to make a definite diagnosis. The following histological classification is oversimplified but workable. There are five main histological categories (Fig. 21.1):

Q12 What do you know about minimal change nephropathy (MCN)?

This only presents with nephrotic syndrome and is the most common cause of nephrotic syndrome in children. It is usually idiopathic, but may rarely

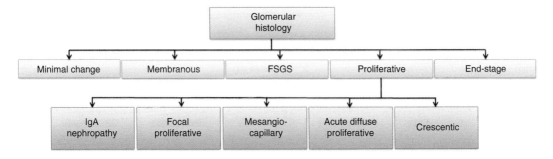

Fig. 21.1 The five main histological categories of glomerulonephritis and five causes of proliferative GN

complicate lymphoma. Glomeruli look normal on light microscopy but show fusion of epithelial foot processes on EM. MCN usually remits completely with prednisolone 1 mg/kg/day given for around 4 weeks, through relapses do occur. Details of this and other treatment regimens are given in the KDIGO Clinical Practice Guideline for Glomerulonephritis (references at the end of this chapter). MCN hardly, if ever, cases renal failure.

Q13 What do you know about membranous nephropathy?

This is the most common cause of the nephrotic syndrome in adults. Usually idiopathic but can be caused by drugs, SLE or malignancy, in up to 20 % of cases. The outcome is best described by the rule of thirds: one third get bet-

ter, one third stay the same and one third get worse. Management is usually supportive though treatment with steroids and cyclophosphamide alternating each month (Ponticelli regimen) may be indicated in severe cases of idiopathic membranous nephropathy with deteriorating renal function and heavy proteinuria (Fig. 21.2).

Q14 What do you know about focal segmental glomerulosclerosis (FSGS)?

This causes proteinuria or nephrotic syndrome and is idiopathic in most cases. Treatment is supportive unless FSGS presents with nephrotic syndrome in which case prednisolone is indicated, though it may need to be used for up to 6 months in order to obtain a remission. Those who relapse as their steroids are tailed down may respond to

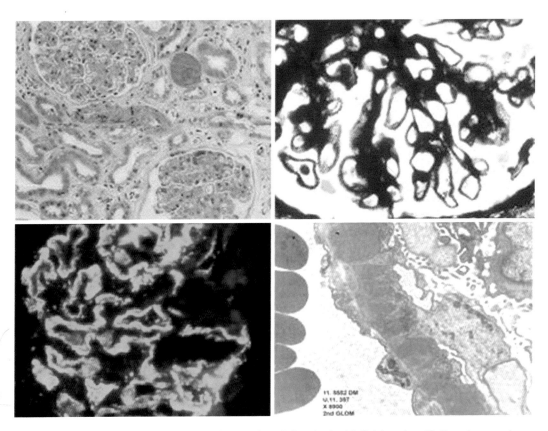

Fig. 21.2 Histology of membranous GN. Microscopic examination shows diffuse thickening of the basement membrane on light microscopy (*top left panel*), with the appearance of "spikes" on silver staining (*top right*) granular deposition of IgG on immunofluorescence (*bottom left*) and subepithelial deposits of IgG on electron microscopy (*bottom right*) – the cause of the thickened basement membrane (Images courtesy of Dr David Kipgen, MRCPath)

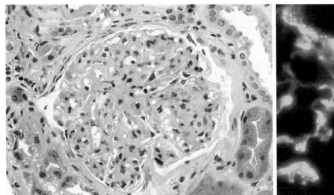 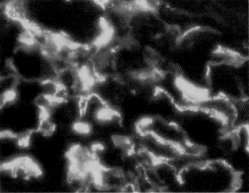

Fig. 21.3 Renal biopsy shows a mesangioproliferative GN with mesangial deposition of IgA on immunofluorescence (Images courtesy of Dr David Kipgen, MRCPath)

the addition of ciclosporin. Up to 50 % of patients with FSGS develop end-stage renal failure within 10 years.

Q15 What do you know about IgA nephropathy?

IgA nephropathy is the commonest cause of GN in the UK. It classically causes recurrent visible (macroscopic) haematuria in young adults, often precipitated by upper respiratory tract infections. Persistent non-visible (microscopic) haematuria may also occur. The cause is unknown though the disease may cluster in families (see Fig. 21.3). Treatment is supportive and outcome is variable. Slow progression to end-stage renal disease occurs in up to 50 % of patients often over 20–25 years of observation. A few will present with severe hypertension, nephrotic range proteinuria and rapidly progressive renal failure. Most of the remaining patients enter a sustained clinical remission or have persistent low-grade hematuria and/or proteinuria.

Note that the haematuria of IgA nephropathy is usually easy to distinguish from the haematuria of acute nephritis. In IgA nephropathy the haematuria occurs immediately after the sore throat and the patient is usually well. In acute nephritis the haematuria occurs 10–14 days after the sore throat and the patient is usually unwell.

Q16 What do you know about focal proliferative GN, mesangiocapillary GN and diffuse proliferative GN?

These are all less common. Focal proliferative GN usually presents with proteinuria, microscopic haematuria and impaired renal function. It is often seen in patients with systemic disease e.g. SLE and SBE. Mesangiocapillary GN is also known as membranoproliferative GN. It causes proteinuria or nephrotic syndrome with microscopic haematuria. Aetiology is unknown although there is an association with partial lipodystrophy in MCGN Type 2. Treatment is supportive. Acute diffuse proliferative GN is the clinical correlate of acute nephritis. It classically occurs 10–14 days after a Streptococcal sore throat or other infection. Treatment is supportive.

Q17 What is meant by "supportive" treatment?

The NICE CKD guideline suggests a target SBP 120–139 mmHg with DBP <90 mmg for patients with CKD and lower targets still if patients have diabetes or urine PCR >100 mg/mmol. Our experience is that SBP 120–129 mmHg is not always achievable, also that aggressive BP reduction is rarely tolerated in the elderly in whom a systolic BP of 150 mmHg is perhaps a reasonable compromise. ACE inhibitors or angiotensin receptor blockers are preferred as first line therapy because of their anti-proteinuric effect. Loop diuretics may be required for patients with oedema due to nephrotic syndrome. Vascular disease is the commonest cause of death in patients with renal failure, and statins have been shown to reduce vascular events in CKD3. Patients with nephrotic syndrome not infrequently have serum cholesterol >8 mmol/l, with many requiring lipid lowering therapy. There is no good evidence that protein restriction will slow the decline in renal function of patients with glomerular disease. Instead an adequate calorie intake with 1 g protein/kg dry body weight plus 1 g protein for every 100 mg/mmol proteinuria is recommended.

Box 21.4 Five supportive treatments for glomerular disease
1. Tight blood pressure control
2. ACEI/ARB for their antiproteinuric effect
3. Loop diuretics for oedema of nephrotic syndrome
4. Statins for hyperlipidaemia
5. Adequate protein/calorie intake to prevent under-nutrition

---

21.1 Objectives: Glomerular Disease

After reading this chapter, you should be able to answer the following:

Q1 What does the term glomerular disease mean?

Q2 Describe the pathophysiology of glomerular disease

Q3 How might you classify glomerular disease?

Q4 How does glomerular disease present?

Q5 What is meant by asymptomatic urinary abnormalities?

Q6 What do you understand by the term acute nephritis?

Q7 What do you understand by the term nephrotic syndrome?

Q8 What is meant by rapidly progressive renal failure?

Q9 Some patients with glomerular disease present with chronic renal failure. How would you make a diagnosis?

Q10 What are the causes of glomerular disease?

Q11 Describe the histological features of glomerular disease.

Q12 What do you know about minimal change nephropathy (MCN)?

Q13 What do you know about membranous nephropathy?

Q14 What do you know about focal segmental glomerular sclerosis (FSGS)?

Q15 What do you know about IgA nephropathy?

Q16 What do you know about focal proliferative GN, mesangiocapillary GN and diffuse proliferative GN?

Q17 What is meant by "supportive" treatment?

Further Reading

1. Chronic Kidney Disease (partial update). Early identification and management of chronic kidney disease in adults in primary and secondary care. National Institute for health and Care Excellence (NICE), Clinical Guideline 182. July 2014.
2. Kidney Disease: Improving Global Outcomes (KDIGO) Glomerulonephritis Work Group. KDIGO Clinical Practice Guideline for Glomerulonephritis. Kidney Inter Suppl. 2012;2:139–274.

Q1 Describe the two types of diabetes and discuss the ways in which they differ.

Type 1 diabetes results from insulin deficiency, with usual onset in teenage or young adult life. It is around ten times less common than type 2 diabetes. Type 2 diabetes is a disease of the middle aged in whom it is usually a consequence of obesity. Far from being insulin deficient, these patients have high levels of insulin in their blood stream which is ineffective because they are overweight. This is known as insulin resistance. Type 2 diabetes can also be a consequence of steroid therapy, for example after renal transplantation. New onset diabetes after transplantation (NODAT) is associated with a high risk of vascular disease. Other types of diabetes that are recognised more often than before are Latent Autoimmune diabetes of Adulthood (LADA) and Maturity Onset Diabetes of the Young (MODY). LADA patients are not always overweight and may progress more rapidly to insulin therapy than is usual in type 2 diabetes, while MODY is a form of diabetes that develops before the age of 25 and does not always require treatment with insulin (Fig. 22.1).

Q2 Describe the complications of diabetes

These are usually considered under two headings – microvascular and macrovascular as shown in the diagram. Diabetes accounts for 1 in 7 of all deaths in the UK. The majority of these are cardiovascular. Diabetes is also the commonest cause of CKD in the UK (Fig. 22.2).

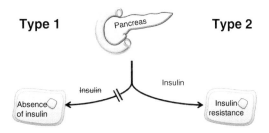

Fig. 22.1 Insulin is required at a cellular level to permit glucose into most cells. Without this process, diabetes occurs. There are only two ways this can happen: (1) Insulin is not produced by the pancreas (*left side*), and so cannot act on the cellular receptors or (2) Insulin *is* produced (often at high levels), but the cells are resistant to its effects (*right side*). The left is type 1 diabetes, and the right type 2

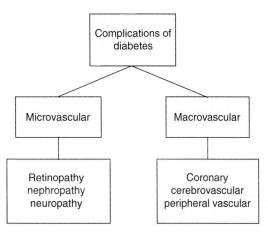

Fig. 22.2 Complications of diabetes

M. Findlay, C. Isles, *Clinical Companion in Nephrology*,
DOI 10.1007/978-3-319-14868-7_22, © Springer International Publishing Switzerland 2015

Fig. 22.3 Progression of proteinuria in diabetes

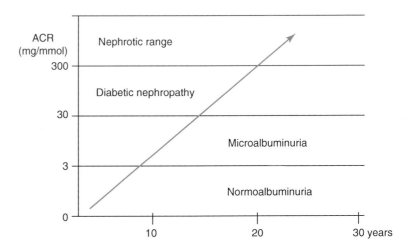

Progression of proteinuria in diabetes

ACR (mg/mmol)

Nephrotic range

300

Diabetic nephropathy

30

Microalbuminuria

3

Normoalbuminuria

0

10   20   30 years

Q3   What do you understand by the term diabetic nephropathy?

Diabetic nephropathy is the classic cause of CKD in people with diabetes. It occurs in up to 40 % of patients after 15–20 years and is more common in those with poor glucose control. It is as likely to occur in type 2 diabetes after 15–20 years though the risk to the individual is greater in type 1 diabetes because type 1 s generally have the disease for longer. The clinical hallmark of diabetic nephropathy is proteinuria and the pathological hallmark is glomerulosclerosis. Figure 22.3 shows how diabetic proteinuria may evolve over a number of years.

Q4   Do all patients with diabetes and renal impairment have diabetic nephropathy?

The triad of diabetes with proteinuria and retinopathy means that the renal disease is almost certainly due to diabetic nephropathy. Most patients with type 1 diabetes who develop proteinuria will have diabetic nephropathy. By contrast, patients with type 2 diabetes and renal impairment often have little or no proteinuria (urine PCR <100 mg/mmol). This type of diabetic renal disease is seen particularly on those who have hypertension and vascular disease at other sites. This is probably due to narrowing of the small arteries in the kidney, so-called hypertensive nephrosclerosis (see Chap. 23).

It is also true that up to 50 % of type 2 diabetics who do have proteinuria will have other forms of proteinuric nephropathy such as FSGS, membranous nephropathy or minimal change disease. In clinical practice this is unlikely to influence management unless nephrotic syndrome is present, raising the possibility that steroids (minimal change and FSGS) or steroids and cyclophosphamide (membranous nephropathy) may be indicated. For these reasons it is not common practice to biopsy a patient with type 2 diabetes and proteinuria unless nephrotic syndrome is present (Fig. 22.4).

Q5   What can be done to slow the rate of progression to renal failure in patients with diabetic nephropathy?

It is generally agreed that the most effective approach is one that addresses multiple risk factors simultaneously. Glucose, proteinuria, hypertension and hyperlipidaemia all provide treatment targets as do lifestyle measures that encourage patients to stop smoking, lose weight and take more exercise.

Q6   How tightly should we control glucose in CKD?

The evidence suggests that good glucose control may prevent diabetic nephropathy but that it has little or no effect on disease progression once proteinuria has been established. The latest KDOQI

Fig. 22.4 Presentations of renal disease in diabetes by degree of proteinuria

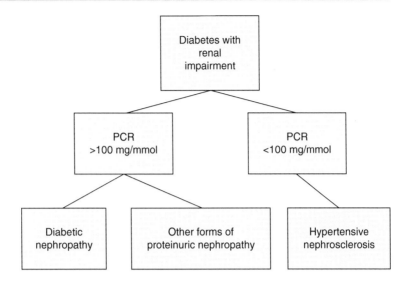

Table 22.1 Conversion guidance for HbA1c

HbA1c (mmol/mol)	HbA1c (%)
42	6.0
48	6.5
53	7.0
58	7.5
64	8.0
75	9.0

guidelines recommend a target hemoglobin A1c (HbA1c) of <53 mmol/mol (<7.0 %) to prevent or delay progression of the microvascular complications of diabetes, including CKD, while quite sensibly suggesting that target HbA1c be extended above 7.0 % in individuals with co-morbidities, limited life expectancy or risk of hypoglycemia. Table 22.1 shows how to convert HbA1c % (previous units) to mmol/mol (current units).

Q7 How should hypertension be managed in diabetes with CKD?

Most people with diabetes and CKD have hypertension, the severity of which predicts the rate of decline of renal function. ACE inhibitors and ARBs have an antiproteinuric effect and have been shown to slow the progression from microalbuminuria to proteinuria to kidney failure in both type 1 and type 2 diabetes. The currently recommended systolic BP target of 130 mmHg is a demanding one and may require not only a highly motivated patient but also up to four or five antihypertensive

drugs. Regular monitoring of renal function is necessary to identify those patients whose GFR falls (hypertensive nephrosclerosis) rather than improves (diabetic nephropathy).

Q8 When should statins be given to patients with diabetes and CKD?

Statins are more likely to reduce the risk of vascular disease in patients with diabetes and CKD than they are to reduce proteinuria or progression to dialysis. The latest guidelines recommend statins to reduce risk of major atherosclerotic events in patients with diabetes and CKD, including those who have received a kidney transplant. Three randomized trials have failed to show benefits for statins in patients with diabetes who are already on dialysis which has led the guideline writers to recommend not initiating statins in this patient subgroup.

Q9 What is the ALPHABET strategy?

This is a useful way of remembering all the things you need to check when you are reviewing a patient with diabetes at the clinic:

Box 22.1 The ALPHABET Strategy
A = Advice on lifestyle especially smoking, diet and exercise.
B = Systolic blood pressure <120–139 mmHg (may accept <140 mmHg)

C = Cholesterol with a target of <4 mmol/l (may accept <5 mmol/l).

D = Diabetes control aiming for HbA1c <53 mmol/mol (may accept <64 mmol/mol)

E = Eye tests which should be annual.

F = Foot care which means annual foot screening as a minimum to risk assess

G = Guardian drugs i.e. guarding against heart disease by giving aspirin & statins when indicated

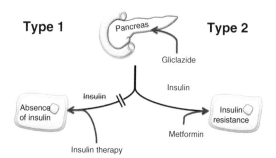

Fig. 22.5 Treatment of diabetes. In type 1 diabetes, insulin must be replaced in order to allow cells to take up and use glucose. In type 2 diabetes, where insulin resistance is the problem, therapy is aimed at increasing the available insulin from the pancreas (gliclazide) or increasing the sensitivity of the tissues to insulin's effects (metformin)

Q10   Discuss the use of sulphonylureas and metformin in diabetic patients with renal disease.

Gliclazide is a sulphonylurea which acts by stimulating the release of insulin from the pancreas. It is probably the most commonly used oral hypoglycaemic in renal patients. The dose range is 40 mg once daily to 160 mg twice daily and the only significant side effects are hypoglycaemia and weight gain. Metformin belongs to a class of drugs called the biguanides and works by increasing the uptake of insulin in peripheral tissues, also by suppressing appetite. Unfortunately metformin is contraindicated in patients with significant renal impairment whose serum creatinine is >200 μmol/l because of the risk of lactic acidosis. Some guidelines recommend withdrawing metformin when serum creatinine exceeds 132 umol/l because of this risk, though we believe the risk is not that high, also that metformin is a very useful drug, and for this reason we have adopted a more relaxed approach to its use. We would however recommend that metformin be stopped temporarily in patients at risk of AKI, for example people with diabetes who are given x-ray contrast or develop diarrhoea.

Q11   Discuss the use of insulin in people who have diabetes and renal disease.

All people with type 1 diabetes will require insulin, as will those type 2 s whose HbA1c cannot be controlled satisfactorily with oral hypoglycaemic drugs. Insulin requirements drop when a patient develops end stage renal failure and starts dialysis. This is because the kidney normally metabolises insulin and does so less efficiently when it is failing. The main advances in insulin therapy in recent years have been the very rapid onset short acting insulins such as novorapid and humalog and the move towards insulin pumps for patients with type 1 diabetes. These advances have increased the options available to patients who require insulin (Fig. 22.5).

Q12   Diabetic patients with renal impairment are more likely to experience hypoglycaemia. Why?

The kidney metabolises 30–40 % of insulin (discussed in Chap. 1 and mentioned above) and also provides up to 45 % of endogenous glucose through gluconeogenesis during prolonged fasting. As a result, patients with diabetes and renal failure are more likely to become hypoglycaemic.

Q13   What other drugs may be used to treat hyperglycaemia?

Patients whose diabetes cannot be controlled with sulphonylureas and who cannot take metformin because of their renal impairment must decide either to try insulin or one of a bewildering array of non insulin alternatives. Five other groups of drugs are available but all have limitations in patients with renal disease. These are the thiazolidinediones, glucagon-like peptide-1 (GLP1) analogues, dipeptidyl peptidate-4 (DPP4) antagonists, sodium-glucose cotransporter 2 (SGLT2) inhibitors and

Fig. 22.6 The incretin system

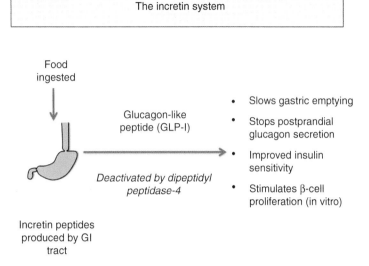

meglitinides. The actions of two of these classes of drugs are outlined above. Incretins, e.g. glucagon-like-peptide, are gut derived hormones secreted in response to nutrient ingestion to promote a number of metabolically beneficial responses, as shown in Fig. 22.6. Two GLP1 analogues and several DPP4 inhibitors are now available for use in the UK, though none have a licence for patients with advanced renal failure. Drugs used to control glycaemia are summarised in Appendix 8.

22.1 Objectives: Renal Disease and Diabetes

After reading this chapter, you should be able to answer the following:

Q1 Describe the two types of diabetes and discuss the ways in which they differ.

Q2 Describe the complications of diabetes.

Q3 What do you understand by the term diabetic nephropathy?

Q4 Do all patients with diabetes and renal impairment have diabetic nephropathy?

Q5 What can be done to slow the rate of progression to renal failure in patients with diabetic nephropathy?

Q6 How tightly should we control glucose in CKD?

Q7 How should hypertension be managed in diabetes with CKD?

Q8 When should statins be given to patients with diabetes and CKD?

Q9 What is the ALPHABET strategy?

Q10 Discuss the use of sulphonylureas and metformin in diabetic patients with renal disease.

Q11 Discuss the use of insulin in people who have diabetes and renal disease.

Q12 Diabetic patients with renal impairment are more likely to experience hypoglycaemia. Why?

Q13 What other drugs may be used to treat hyperglycaemia?

Further Reading

1. National Kidney Foundation KDOQI Clinical Practice Guidelines and Clinical Practice recommendations for Diabetes and Chronic Kidney Disease. AJKD. 2007;49(2 Suppl 2):S1–179.
2. National Kidney Foundation. KDOQI Clinical Practice Guideline for Diabetes and CKD: 2012 update. Am J Kidney Dis. 2012;60:850–86.

Q1 What do you understand by the term renovascular disease?

Renovascular disease, sometimes referred to as "ischaemic nephropathy" is a term used to describe patients with narrowing of either their main renal (large vessel) or intra-renal (small vessel) arteries or arterioles.

Q2 How does renovascular disease of the main renal arteries present clinically?

A number of clinical presentations are recognised. Large vessel renovascular disease causes problems when one or more of the main renal arteries are stenosed >60 % as this is the degree of stenosis required to reduce blood flow. Hypertension is an important consequence of both unilateral and bilateral renal artery stenosis. AKI is frequently precipitated by ACE inhibitors in patients with previously unsuspected bilateral disease or stenosis to a single kidney. CKD and cardiorenal failure can also occur in patients with bilateral disease or stenosis to a single kidney (Fig. 23.1).

Q3 How does small vessel renovascular disease present clinically?

Three clinical presentations are recognised. The most common, hypertensive nephrosclerosis, is best thought of as renal artery stenosis affecting the intrarenal arteries. The term malignant hypertension describes a severe form of hypertension with diastolic pressure usually >130 mmHg, bilateral retinal haemorrhages and exudates and/or bilateral papilloedema. The histological hallmark is fibrinoid necrosis of the intrarenal arterioles. Atheroembolism (aka cholesterol embolism) occurs when cholesterol crystals break off from an atheromatous aortic wall to be swept downstream to the kidneys and peripheral vessels. Those that lodge in the kidneys do so in small arterioles where they provoke a fibrotic

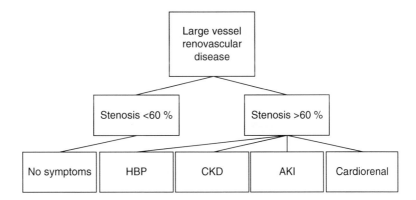

Fig. 23.1 Presentation of large vessel renovascular disease

M. Findlay, C. Isles, *Clinical Companion in Nephrology*,
DOI 10.1007/978-3-319-14868-7_23, © Springer International Publishing Switzerland 2015

reaction which eventually occludes the lumen of these vessels causing subacute renal failure (2 or 3 weeks after the insult rather than 2 or 3 days). We report a case below. Diagnosis of atheroembolism can be made without a renal biopsy if the following triad is present:

- A precipitating factor such as aortic instrumentation e.g. coronary angiography.
- Subacute renal failure (as above).
- Peripheral embolisation causing a livedo reticularis over the knees and the so-called purple toe syndrome.

Case Report

A 66 year old man presented with subacute renal failure, livedo reticularis and purple toes 2 months after coronary angiography. This was on a background of hypertension, previous inferior MI, peripheral vascular disease and an abdominal aortic aneurysm. Renal function had been normal at the time of coronary angiography. Renal biopsy identified elongated bi-convex needle shaped cholesterol crystals occluding the lumen of a small artery (see Fig. 23.2). This patient's course was complicated by severe acute pancreatitis (a recognised complication of atheroembolism) which led to multi organ failure requiring dialysis, ventilation and inotropic support. He

---

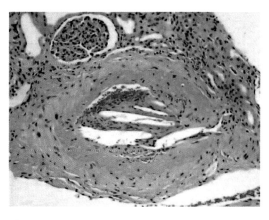

Fig. 23.2 Case report of cholesterol emboli with histological section demonstrating cholesterol emboli within renal arteriole

---

remained dialysis dependent for 35 months before eventually recovering enough renal function to stop renal replacement therapy.

Cuddy E et al. Risk of coronary angiography. *Lancet.* 2005;366:182; with permission from Elsevier

---

Q4 What causes renovascular disease of the main renal arteries?

There are two main causes:

1. Atherosclerotic renovascular disease (ARVD). This accounts for >90 % cases. ARVD is a disease of the middle aged and elderly, commonly associated with smoking, diabetes and vascular disease at other sites. As such it should be managed with appropriate secondary prevention.

2. Fibromuscular dysplasia (FMD) accounts for the remainder. This is a disorder of (mostly) females commonly affecting renal and arteries of the head and neck. FMD more commonly affects a younger cohort than ARVD

Q5 Why do patients with renovascular disease become hypertensive?

There are thought to be two main mechanisms. Stenosis >60 % of a main renal artery will cause reduction in renal perfusion which stimulates the renin angiotensin system leading in turn to high circulating levels of angiotensin II (which has a direct pressor effect on blood vessels) and aldosterone (which causes sodium retention).

Q6 When should you suspect renovascular disease?

It is worth considering a diagnosis of renovascular disease and possibly undertaking further investigations in the following circumstances:

Box 23.1 Think Renovascular If

- Hypertension is severe or of recent onset
- Kidneys are asymmetrical in size
- Cardiorenal failure
- Peripheral vascular disease
- ACE inhibitor induced AKI

Q7 How would you confirm a diagnosis of renovascular disease?

You would normally only do so if you thought this was going to influence management. The choice then lies between CT renal angiography and MR angiography. CTRA involves ionising radiation and iodinated contrast medium, and is associated with a risk of contrast nephropathy in patients with eGFR <30 ml/min (see Chap. 10). It is reasonably good at ruling out (sensitivity 59–96 %) and ruling in (specificity 82–99 %) haemodynamically significant ARVD though false negatives and false positives do occur. MR angiography produces images without radiation or iodinated contrast, although these usually require gadolinium enhancement which carries a risk of nephrogenic systemic fibrosis when eGFR is less than 30 ml/min. MRA has similar diagnostic accuracy to CTRA.

Q8 What do you know about nephrogenic systemic fibrosis?

NSF is a rare disorder with widespread skin and possibly other tissue fibrotic processes in lungs, muscle and heart. The differential diagnosis includes scleroderma. NSF only occurs in AKI or patients with CKD stage 4 and 5 in whom the odds ratio for developing NSF after gadolinium is around 30. There is no known treatment. NSF can be prevented by avoiding gadolinium in patients whose GFR is <30 ml/min.

Q9 What are the treatment options once ARVD has been confirmed?

The options are best medical therapy, renal vascularisation or a combination of the two. Best medical therapy consists of aggressive medical management of hypertension and diabetes if present, along with antiplatelet drugs and a statin to reduce the risk of vascular disease elsewhere. ACE inhibitors might seem a logical choice here but may lead to a significant reduction in GFR in patients with bilateral renal artery stenosis, with unilateral renal artery stenosis and a solitary kidney, and in those with hypertensive nephrosclerosis (intrarenal artery stenosis). This does not contraindicate their use but does emphasise the importance of monitoring renal function and being prepared to stop the drug in the event that GFR falls precipitously. A slight early fall in GFR is common after starting an ACE inhibitor and not a reason to stop the drug whereas a fall in GFR of greater than 25 % should alert the clinician to the possibility of ARVD/hypertensive nephrosclerosis. The good news is that the ACE inhibitor reduction in GFR in renovascular disease almost always resolves after stopping the drug.

Q10 When is renal artery revascularisation indicated?

Rarely. The results of two large randomised trials, ASTRAL and CORAL, have shown that medical therapy without stenting is the preferred management strategy for the majority of patients with atherosclerotic renal-artery stenosis. CORAL only randomised patients with arterial stenosis >60 % and was unable even to show a benefit in the subgroup of patients whose arterial stenosis was >80 %. Only patients whose clinicians were 'uncertain' of the benefits of revascularisation were randomised to these trials so it remains possible that occasional patients will benefit from stenting. These are likely to include patients with cardiorenal failure due to bilateral renovascular disease. Even in this high risk group a watch and wait policy may be just as appropriate as early intervention, as shown by the history below.

Case Report

A 73 year woman presented with pulmonary oedema due to acute coronary syndrome. Serum creatinine was raised at 256 umol/l (eGFR 17 ml/min). Both kidneys were 8 cm in bipolar diameter and CT renal angiogram showed 87 % left and 82 % right renal artery stenosis. We did not randomize her to ASTRAL because we were convinced she would benefit from stenting while she declined both coronary angiography and renal revascularization as she was certain that neither were necessary. She subsequently did well for 4 years with

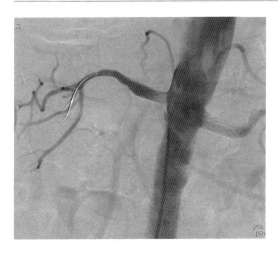

Fig. 23.3 Image of right renal artery following percutaneous angioplasty and stenting

serum creatinine 160–180 umol/l until presenting again with pulmonary oedema and AKI. Two weeks of dialysis dependence followed before she was fit enough for further renal angiography which confirmed tight bilateral ostial stenosis. She began to diurese within 24 h of stenting (Fig. 23.3) and has not required further dialysis during 42 months of follow up. She has since developed AF with mild congestive failure, well controlled on digoxin and frusemide. Her most recent BP was 140/72 mmHg with serum creatinine 149 umol/l (eGFR 30 ml/min).

Li WS et al. Bilateral renovascular disease with cardiorenal failure: intervene early or watch and wait? QJM. 2012;105:567–9; with permission from Oxford University Press.

23.1 Objectives: Renovascular Disease

After reading this chapter you should be able to answer the following:

Q1 What do you understand by the term renovascular disease?

Q2 How does renovascular disease of the main renal arteries present clinically?

Q3 How does small vessel renovascular disease present clinically?

Q4 What causes renovascular disease in the main renal arteries?

Q5 Why do patients with renovascular disease become hypertensive?

Q6 When should you suspect renovascular disease?

Q7 How would you confirm a diagnosis of renovascular disease?

Q8 What do you know about nephrogenic systemic fibrosis?

Q9 What are the treatment options once ARVD has been confirmed?

Q10 When is renal artery revascularisation indicated?

Further Reading

1. Cooper C, et al. Stenting and medical therapy for atherosclerotic renal artery stenosis. N Engl J Med. 2014;370:13–22.

This chapter is primarily concerned with the diagnosis, investigation and management of hypertension generally, though many of the questions and answers are relevant to patients with CKD too.

Q1 What do you understand by the terms systolic and diastolic blood pressure?

Blood pressure is the term used to describe the pressure that exists within the main arteries. This is written as systolic/diastolic e.g. 120/80 mmHg. Systolic blood pressure is best thought of as the pressure in the main arteries with each heart contraction, and diastolic pressure the pressure in the main arteries when the heart is relaxing.

Q2 Define hypertension.

Hypertension is that level of blood pressure at which the benefits of treatment outweigh the risks. In those with kidney disease, heart disease, previous stroke or diabetes, the level at which benefits outweigh risks of treatment and is thought to be around 140/90 mmHg. For younger patients at low risk who have nothing else wrong e.g. a young woman who does not smoke, have high cholesterol or a family history of premature vascular disease it may be acceptable to monitor BP in the range 140/90–160/100 without drug treatment (see later).

Q3 What is meant by the term isolated systolic hypertension?

Isolated systolic hypertension means a systolic pressure >140 mmHg and a diastolic pressure <90 mmHg. This is a common finding in older patients, including those on dialysis, and is likely to reflect the fact that they have stiffer arteries than younger people.

Q4 Discuss how you might use clinic BP, home blood pressure monitoring (HBPM) & ambulatory blood pressure monitoring (ABPM) to make a diagnosis of hypertension.

The NICE 2011 guideline on hypertension recommends greater use of ambulatory and home monitoring to confirm the diagnosis of hypertension. ABPM is still probably the gold standard but HBPM is a suitable alternative and certainly more convenient for the patient (Fig. 24.1).

Q5 What risks are associated with hypertension?

Hypertension increases the risk of heart attack and stroke by a factor of 2–4. Hypertensive patients are more likely to present with heart failure and to have peripheral vascular disease including abdominal aortic aneurysms. Patients whose diastolic pressure is greater than 130 mmHg may develop a condition called malignant hypertension, particularly if the rate of rise of their blood pressure is very rapid. Malignant hypertension is characterised by headaches and visual blurring, is associated with retinal haemorrhages, exudates and papilloedema, and can also cause renal failure. In countries such as South Africa malignant hypertension is the commonest cause of kidney disease requiring dialysis (Fig. 24.2).

M. Findlay, C. Isles, *Clinical Companion in Nephrology*,
DOI 10.1007/978-3-319-14868-7_24, © Springer International Publishing Switzerland 2015

Fig. 24.1 NICE guideline recommendation for confirmation of hypertension

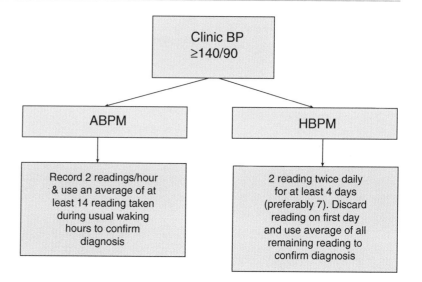

both his salt and alcohol intake. Kidney patients should be advised not to buy Lo-Salt in the belief that this will be better for them than ordinary salt. Lo-Salt contains potassium chloride, and while there is some evidence that this might lower blood pressure slightly, the risks of hyperkalaemia far outweigh the benefits. Stopping smoking will not lower blood pressure but will reduce risk of heart attack and stroke by other means. Patients whose blood pressure remains high despite lifestyle measures will require drug therapy.

Q7 What level of blood pressure would you recommend antihypertensive drug treatment?

The NICE 2011 guideline recommends starting antihypertensive drug treatment immediately if clinic BP ≥180/110 mmHg. If clinic BP is less than this then NICE suggest that the decision on drug treatment should be based on the results of ABPM/HBPM, the patients age and the presence or absence of target organ damage and other risk factors as shown below (Fig. 24.3):

Q8 How does Clinic BP relate to Ambulatory or Home BP?

Ambulatory and home readings are systematically lower than clinic readings, which means you should start drug therapy at lower levels of pressure if using ambulatory or home readings. The relation between clinic and ABPM/HBPM is shown (Fig. 24.4).

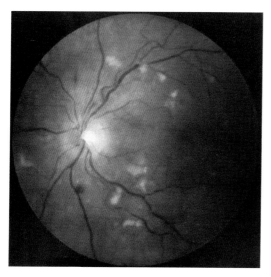

Fig. 24.2 Hypertensive retinopathy as seen on fundoscopy showing flame haemorrhages, "cotton wool" spots and papilloedema

Q6 What lifestyle measures have been shown to lower blood pressure?

The lifestyles measures that have been shown to reduce blood pressure include weight reduction if obese, salt restriction to a pinch of salt in cooking with none at table, and restriction of alcohol intake to less than 2 or 3 units per day. An overweight, heavy drinking hypertensive patient who adds small handfuls of salt to his food might expect to drop his systolic blood pressure by 5–10 mmHg by losing weight and restricting

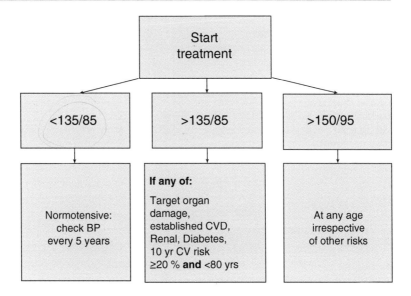

Fig. 24.3 Thresholds for pharmacological control of blood pressure

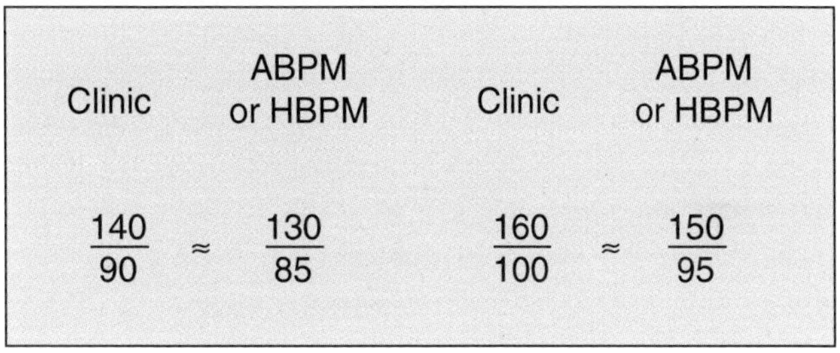

Fig. 24.4 Approximation of clinic against ABPM/HBPM reading

Q9 What drug therapies are available to treat hypertension?

Six classes of antihypertensive drugs are commonly used to treat hypertension. These can be remembered by using the ABCD mnemonic as follows:

- A = ACE inhibitor, Angiotensin receptor blocker, Alpha-blocker
- B = Beta-blocker
- C = Calcium channel blocker
- D = Diuretic

Q10 Which antihypertensive drug would you give to a patient who did not have kidney disease?

We summarise the recommendations made by NICE in their 2011 Guideline in Fig. 24.5. Our own practice differs only slightly. When prescribing prescribing a diuretic, NICE recommend a thiazide like diuretic such as chlorthalidone or indapamide rather than a thiazide. We and others

have continued to use bendroflumethiazide 2.5 mg once daily as first line diuretic in patients with hypertension.

Q11 In what way would this advice differ for a patient with chronic kidney disease?

The short answer is that ACE inhibitors and ARBs have been shown to be renoprotective in patients with proteinuric nephropathy. It is of course more complicated than this as opinion differs on the level of proteinuria required for this diagnosis. The American KDIGO guideline suggests that ACE inhibitors or ARBs be used when urine ACR >3 mg/mmol while others have adopted a more conservative approach and only prescribe ACE inhibitors and ARBs for their renoprotective effect when urine ACR >30 mg/mmol (which is roughly the same as PCR >50 mg/mmol for those who use PCR). These drugs are frequently associated with a small rise in serum creatinine when first given to patients

Fig. 24.5 NICE recommendation for BP control. *A* ACEi or ARB, *C* calcium channel blocker, *D* thiazide like diuretic, *CCB preferred but consider thiazide-like diuretic (TLD) with oedema or HF, °consider low dose spironolactone or higher doses of TLD

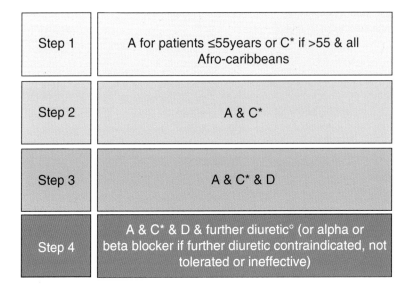

Step 1	A for patients ≤55years or C* if >55 & all Afro-caribbeans
Step 2	A & C*
Step 3	A & C* & D
Step 4	A & C* & D & further diuretic° (or alpha or beta blocker if further diuretic contraindicated, not tolerated or ineffective)

with CKD, though this is not normally a reason to stop: many nephrologists will tolerate a rise in serum creatinine of up to 30 % or a fall in eGFR of up to 25 % before doing so. ACE inhibitors and ARBs may also increase serum potassium because they lower serum aldosterone. These drugs should not be started if serum K is greater than 5 mmol/l and should be stopped if serum K goes over 6 mmol/l. So far as the other antihypertensive drugs are concerned, thiazides become less effective as antihypertensive agents when serum creatinine exceeds 150 μmol/l, in which case patients should normally be given a loop diuretic such as frusemide if a diuretic is required to control blood pressure. There are no particular advantages or disadvantages to giving calcium channel blockers, alpha-blockers or beta-blockers to patients with CKD.

Q12 How should you monitor blood pressure treatment and what level of blood pressure should you aim for?

NICE recommend clinic blood pressure measurements to monitor the response to drug treatment unless the patient has been shown to have a white coat effect, that is a discrepancy of more than 20/10 mmHg between clinic and average day time ambulatory pressure or average home

pressure measurements at the time of diagnosis, in which case ABPM or HBPM should be used together with clinic blood pressure measurements to monitor the response to treatment. Target clinic pressure when CKD is not present is below 140/90 mmHg for those under 80 years and below 150/90 mmHg in people aged 80 years and over. For target BP in patients with CKD see Q17, Chap. 21.

Q13 What is meant by the term resistant hypertension?

The term resistant hypertension is usually used to describe a patient whose clinic pressure remains higher than 140/90 after treatment with optimal or best tolerated triple therapy. The options at this stage are as follows:

Box 24.1 Options for Managing Resistant Hypertension
1. Check concordance
2. Evaluate for underlying cause
3. Re-emphasise importance of non-drug therapy
4. Consider ABPM/HBPM
5. Add a fourth drug

NICE recommend further diuretic treatment with low dose Spironolactone 25 mg once daily provided serum potassium is not greater than 4.5 mmol/l and with higher dose thiazide-like diuretic treatment if serum potassium is higher than this. We would tend to switch from bendroflumethiazide to frusemide at this point. The starting dose of frusemide is 40 mg once daily but can be increased slowly to 80 mg twice daily if necessary and if tolerated. An alpha-blocker such as doxazosin MR 4 mg once daily or beta-blocker e.g. atenolol 25–100 mg once daily may be given if further diuretic treatment is not tolerated, contraindicated or ineffective.

Q14 What should you tell a patient when starting an antihypertensive drug?

You should say that you are doing so to reduce their risk of heart attack or stroke; that treatment will be lifelong; that hypertensive patients commonly require two, three or four drugs in order to control their pressure as none of the drugs are particularly effective when given alone; that these drugs are generally well tolerated with up to 80 % of patients having no side effects whatsoever; that when side effects do occur these are always reversible and will resolve when the drug is withdrawn. We discuss the side effects of the different antihypertensive drugs in more detail in the next chapter

Q15 What does concordance mean and what steps can you take to improve it?

Concordance is the term used to describe the extent to which a patient is taking his or her drug treatment. Concordance is known to be low in patients who have symptomless conditions such as high blood pressure. Patients are more likely to adhere to antihypertensives if they engage with their physician. This was recognised by the guideline writer who wrote that 'the most gifted physician armed with the most powerful antihypertensive drugs will not control blood pressure unless he or she can engage with the patient'.

24.1 Objectives: Hypertension

After reading this chapter, you should be able to answer the following:

Q1 What do you understand by the terms systolic and diastolic blood pressure?

Q2 Define hypertension.

Q3 What is meant by the term isolated systolic hypertension?

Q4 Discuss how you might use clinic BP, home blood pressure monitoring (HBPM) and ambulatory blood pressure monitoring (ABPM) to make a diagnosis of hypertension.

Q5 What risks are associated with hypertension?

Q6 What lifestyle measures have been shown to lower blood pressure?

Q7 What level of blood pressure would you recommend antihypertensive drug treatment?

Q8 How does Clinic BP relate to Ambulatory or Home BP?

Q9 What drug therapies are available to treat hypertension?

Q10 Which antihypertensive drug would you give to a patient who did not have kidney disease?

Q11 In what way would this advice differ for a patient with chronic kidney disease?

Q12 How should you monitor blood pressure treatment and what level of blood pressure should you aim for?

Q13   What is meant by the term resistant hypertension?

Q14   What should you tell a patient when starting an antihypertensive drug?

Q15   What does concordance mean and what steps can you take to improve it?

Further Reading

1. Hypertension, Clinical management of primary hypertension in adults. National Institute for health and Care Excellence (NICE), Clinical Guideline 127. Aug 2011.
2. Kidney Disease: Improving Global Outcomes (KDIGO) Blood Pressure Working Group. KDIGO Clinical Practice Guideline for the Management of Blood Pressure in Chronic Kidney Disease. Kidney Int Suppl. 2012;2:337–414.

Antihypertensive Drugs

25

Q1 What should you know about ACE inhibitors?

These drugs all end in –pril. Examples are lisinopril, ramipril, perindopril and enalapril. The dose range for lisinopril in hypertension is 5–40 mg once daily. The ACE inhibitors block the conversion of angiotensin 1 to angiotensin II by inhibiting angiotensin converting enzyme. Angiotensin II is a powerful vasoconstrictor and in this way blood pressure is thought to be lowered. ACE inhibitors have antiproteinuric properties and are specifically indicated in patients with proteinuric nephropathy (urine PCR >50 mg/mmol). The commonest side effect of an ACE inhibitor is a dry cough, the occurrence of which should prompt a switch to an angiotensin receptor blocker. We have already alluded to the fact that ACE inhibitors may worsen renal function in patients with bilateral renovascular disease and also cause hyperkalaemia. This is in addition to an acute worsening of renal function if the patient becomes intravascularly deplete. Patients prescribed an ACE inhibitor must be advised to omit this drug and seek help from their general practitioner if they start vomiting or develop diarrhoea in order to reduce the risk of drug induced AKI.

Q2 What should you know angiotensin receptor blockers?

These drugs all end in –sartan. Examples are losartan, irbesartan and valsartan. The dose range for losartan in hypertension is 25–100 mg daily in 1 or 2 divided doses. ARBs lower blood pres-

sure by blocking the receptor to which angiotensin II binds, but do not cause cough. They share an antiproteinuric effect with ACE inhibitors and are also as likely to cause hyperkalaemia, worsen renal function in patients with bilateral renovascular disease and AKI in the context of dehydration. ARBs should not be combined with ACE inhibitors as this may result in more adverse events without any added clinical benefit.

Q3 What should you know calcium channel blockers?

Calcium channel blockers are vasodilators. There are two types: dihydropyridines such as amlodipine and nifedipine which do not lower heart rate, and rate-limiting calcium channel blockers diltiazem and verapamil which do. Amlodipine 5–10 mg once daily is the most commonly prescribed dihydropyridine calcium channel blocker. It is generally well tolerated, is easy to combine with other drugs but can cause troublesome ankle swelling. It is important to avoid co-prescribing a rate limiting calcium channel blocker with a beta blocker, out-with exceptional circumstances, as this can lead to profound bradycardia.

Q4 What should you know about thiazide diuretics?

Bendroflumethiazide 2.5 mg once daily, was and probably still is the diuretic of choice for hypertension. This is despite the NICE recommendation that if a diuretic is to be started or

M. Findlay, C. Isles, *Clinical Companion in Nephrology*,
DOI 10.1007/978-3-319-14868-7_25, © Springer International Publishing Switzerland 2015

changed clinicians should offer a thiazide-like diuretic such as chlorthalidone 12.5–25 mg once daily or indapamide 1.5 mg modified release or 2.5 mg standard preparation once daily instead. NICE do concede that for people already taking bendroflumethiazide whose blood pressure is stable and well controlled, it is acceptable to continue treatment with bendroflumethiazide. Gout and hyponatraemia are two important side effects. Thiazides are more likely to cause hyponatraemia than loop diuretics because they impair free water clearance to a greater extent.

Q5 What should you know about loop diuretics?

Frusemide is the most commonly prescribed loop diuretic. Others in this class are bumetanide and torasemide. The starting dose of frusemide is 40 mg daily. This can normally be increased by increments of 40–80 mg twice daily if necessary and if tolerated. As a general rule larger doses of loop diuretics are required for patients with chronic kidney disease than in those with normal renal function. This is because loop diuretics are pumped into the proximal convoluted tubule by what is known as the common anion secretor pathway, where they have to compete with other anionic substances, the levels of which increase

as kidney function becomes more impaired. Gout is an important side effect.

Q6 Thiazide and loop diuretics frequently cause hypokalaemic alkalosis in patients with normal renal function. Why?

As a result of blocking pumps in the thick ascending limb of the Loop of Henle (loop diuretics) and the distal convoluted tubule (thiazide diuretics) more sodium is delivered distally to the cortical collecting duct. Sodium is exchanged for potassium by the principal cells in the cortical collecting duct while potassium is exchanged for hydrogen ions by the intercalated cell, also in the cortical collecting duct. The result is hypokalaemic alkalosis (see Fig. 25.1).

Q7 What should you know about alpha-blockers?

Alphablockers are vasodilators that act by blocking the alpha receptor on blood vessel walls. The most commonly prescribed alpha-blocker for control of hypertension is doxazosin, the best tolerated preparation of which is doxazosin MR 4 mg once daily. Doxazosin can be added on to any of the other antihypertensive drugs and is not any more likely to cause side effects in a kidney patient than in patients who do not have chronic

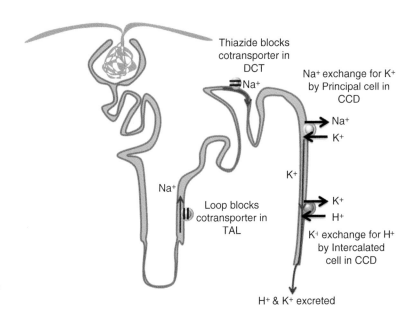

Fig. 25.1 Site of action of loop and thiazide diuretics

kidney disease. Side effects include tiredness, lethargy and dizziness.

Q8   What should you know beta-blockers?

Beta-blockers block beta receptors which are found in many tissues including blood vessels, heart, kidney and lung. Examples are bisoprolol, atenolol and carvedilol. The dose range for bisoprolol in hypertension is 5–20 mg once daily. Beta-blockers probably lower blood pressure by suppressing the release of renin by the kidney and by reducing cardiac output. You can judge whether a patient is beta-blocked or not by checking their pulse, aiming for a heart rate of around 60 per minute. If lower than this then most would not normally use a betablocker. Beta-blockers used to be one of the mainstays of treatment of hypertension but recent trials have suggested they are less effective than calcium channel blockers and ACE inhibitors and as a result of this they are no longer recommended as 1st line therapy. Side effects are common and include cold hands, lethargy and erectile dysfunction. They are contraindicated in patients with asthma, also in COPD if the peak flow rate is less than 300 litres/min.

25.1   Objectives: Antihypertensive Drugs

After reading this chapter, you should be able to answer the following:

Q1   What should you know about ACE inhibitors?

Q2   What should you know angiotensin receptor blockers?

Q3   What should you know calcium channel blockers?

Q4   What should you know about thiazide diuretics?

Q5   What should you know about loop diuretics?

Q6   Thiazide and loop diuretics frequently cause hypokalaemic alkalosis in patients with normal renal function. Why?

Q7   What should you know about alpha-blockers?

Q8   What should you know about beta-blockers?

Further Reading

1. Ashley C, Dunleavy A. The Renal Drug Handbook 4th Edition. Radcliffe Publishing: London, UK; 2014.

Q1 What is ADPKD?

Autosomal dominant polycystic kidney disease is a relatively common (prevalence 1 in 1,000) and important cause of CKD. Eighty-five percent of cases are caused by mutations of the PKD1 gene with the remaining 15 % of cases due to mutations of the PKD2 gene. These mutations cause defective cell signalling which leads to cyst formation. Small cysts develop in childhood but may not be detectable until early adult life.

Q2 How might a patient with polycystic kidney disease present clinically?

Most patients with ADPKD have no symptoms. Some experience loin discomfort and others a fullness in their abdomen. When acute pain occurs this is likely to be due to haemorrhage or infection in a cyst. ADPKD may also come to light during investigation of hypertension, chronic kidney disease or subarachnoid haemorrhage. Although polycystic kidneys are the commonest cause of renal masses that find their way into clinical examinations, some are easier to feel than others which means that on occasion only one and sometimes neither kidney is palpable.

Q3 Describe the extra renal manifestations of polycystic kidneys.

The most important are erythrocytosis, hepatic cyst formation and intracranial aneurysms. Erythrocytosis occurs because the cysts produce erythropoietin. It is usually inferred because patients with polycystic kidney disease are generally less anaemic than you would expect for a given level of renal failure. Hepatic cysts can cause hepatomegaly which may be quite striking, though liver failure is rare. Intracranial aneurysms are said to occur in around 10 % of patients with polycystic kidneys and may bleed causing subarachnoid haemorrhage.

Q4 How is the diagnosis of ADKPD made?

If a patient has a family history of polycystic kidneys, palpable masses in both loins and enlarged kidneys containing multiple cysts on renal ultrasound then the diagnosis is very easy and obvious. Difficulties may arise if there is no family history (possible new mutation), kidneys that are difficult to feel (not uncommon) or an ultrasound report which mentions only a few cysts and does not specify the renal size. Ultrasonic criteria for ADPKD are in fact quite well defined. In a patient with a positive family history then a diagnosis of ADPKD is likely if the kidneys are enlarged (>12 cm) with two or more cysts in one or both kidneys by the age of 30, two or more bilaterally by age 59 and four or more cysts in both kidneys from age 60 onwards (Fig. 26.1).

In order to diagnose ADPKD when there is no family history there must be bilateral cysts in bilaterally enlarged kidneys or the presence of multiple bilateral renal and hepatic cysts. Ultrasound can detect cysts from 1 cm in diameter and is the preferred form of imaging. CT will show cysts as small as 0.5 cm but exposes the patient to radiation (Fig. 26.2). MR is an equally sensitive alternative to CT.

M. Findlay, C. Isles, *Clinical Companion in Nephrology*,
DOI 10.1007/978-3-319-14868-7_26, © Springer International Publishing Switzerland 2015

Fig. 26.1 Ultrasound criteria for diagnosis of ADPKD type 1 in those with positive family history

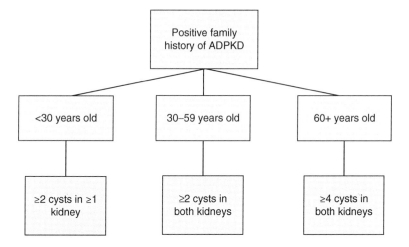

any benefits from current treatments. A negative scan at 20 is falsely negative in 4 % of cases which means that further scanning will be necessary in order to exclude the disease with certainty. We normally recommend that this is undertaken at age of 30 by which time the false negative rate for ultrasound scanning is very nearly zero.

Q6 What is the role of genetic testing in ADPKD?

Limited. Genetic screening is available in specialist centres only. It requires several affected family members to be tested but is not generally recommended as it hardly ever alters management. It might be used to determine whether it would be safe for the child of an affected parent to donate a kidney but otherwise it is of limited value as it does not, for example, predict the time that renal function will begin to deteriorate or the ultimate severity of the disease.

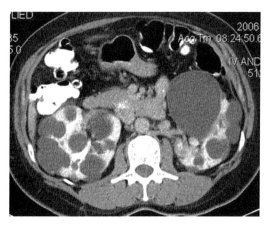

Fig. 26.2 Abdominal CT showing multiple cysts of varying size in both kidneys consistent with autosomal dominant polycystic kidney disease. The diagnosis is usually made with ultrasound but the cysts are more easily seen on CT

Q5 Whom and when to screen?

The inheritance of polycystic kidney disease presenting in adulthood is autosomal dominant which means that 50 % of the offspring of an affected parent will have the abnormal gene and develop cysts in both kidneys. Screening those under the age of 20 is not routinely recommended for two reasons: practically, because the cysts grow slowly and may not be visible on ultrasound in childhood and adolescence and, perhaps more importantly, because the risks of labelling a young person with this diagnosis – with potential psychological damage and implications to education and career – are not currently outweighed by

Q7 Does the presence of multiple renal cysts always mean that a patient has ADPKD?

No. Simple renal cysts are common and may be multiple though renal size will be normal and there will be no family history of ADPKD in such patients. Autosomal recessive polycystic kidney disease (ARPKD) is fortunately very rare as it causes renal failure in childhood. Juvenile nephronophthisis (aka medullary cystic disease) is an autosomal recessive disorder that leads to multiple small cysts throughout both kidneys and progressive renal failure in adolescence.

Medullary sponge kidney is a congenital disorder characterised by tiny cysts in the medullary collecting ducts. It is associated with stone formation but not usually with renal failure. Multiple renal cysts can also develop in patients who have had their kidney disease for many years, especially those who are on renal replacement therapy. This is known as acquired cystic kidney disease or ACKD and is harmless.

Q8 Discuss the management and outcome of polycystic kidney disease.

The only treatment option currently available is control of blood pressure which is commonly raised in polycystic kidney disease. ACE inhibitors are usually recommended as first-line therapy though it is by no means certain that they have advantages over other antihypertensive drugs, and anyway most patients require more than one drug to achieve clinic blood pressure that is consistently less than 140/90. Blood pressure apart, there is currently nothing else that can be done to halt the progression of kidney failure once renal function has begun to decline. Patients may be told that it takes about 10 years to reach dialysis from the moment the creatinine begins to rise, also that the average age at which dialysis is required is around 50 for patients who carry the PKD1 gene and 70 for those with ADPKD type 2. This effectively means that many patients with the milder form of the disease will not require dialysis during their lifetime.

Q9 When is surgery indicated in ADPKD?

Not very often. Aspiration of large cysts under ultrasound or CT guidance may be of value if these are causing pain. Laparoscopic or surgical cyst defenestration may be indicated if multiple cysts are causing pain. Nephrectomy is reserved for recurrent life-threatening infection, bleeding, renal cancer (which when it occurs is more often bilateral in ADPKD), and in cases where the kidneys are so large that they would interfere with placement of a renal transplant.

26.1 Objectives: Polycystic Kidney Disease

After reading this chapter, you should be able to answer the following:

Q1 What is ADPKD?

Q2 How might a patient with polycystic kidney disease present clinically?

Q3 Describe the extra renal manifestations of polycystic kidneys.

Q4 How is the diagnosis of ADKPD made?

Q5 Whom and when to screen?

Q6 What is the role of genetic testing in ADPKD?

Q7 Does the presence of multiple renal cysts always mean that a patient has ADPKD?

Q8 Discuss the management and outcome of polycystic kidney disease.

Q9 When is surgery indicated in ADPKD?

Further Reading

1. Torres VE, et al. Autosomal dominant polycystic kidney disease. Lancet. 2007;369:1287–301.

Anaemia is a common problem in chronic kidney disease and is associated with considerable morbidity and mortality if untreated. During the past few years effective treatment has become possible with genetically engineered erythropoiesis stimulating agents (ESAs) and intravenous iron.

Q1 What is haemoglobin and what are the normal levels?

Haemoglobin is the part of the red blood cell that carries oxygen to the tissues. Normal range for men is 135–180 g/l and women 120–160 g/l. Mildly low levels are particularly common in women. In general the body adapts well to mild chronic anaemia, causing few, if any, symptoms.

Q2 Why do patients with CKD become anaemic?

There are a number of reasons. The main one is lack of erythropoietin but a reduced red cell life span, iron deficiency, drugs and procedures also contribute (Fig. 27.1):

Q3 What are the symptoms of anaemia?

Tiredness, lack of energy, breathlessness on exertion, poor appetite, poor concentration, disturbed and un-refreshing sleep are all symptoms of anaemia. Symptoms are very similar to those of uraemia and indeed anaemia may be the cause of these. The presence of anaemia may worsen or unmask angina if patients have underlying ischaemic heart disease, due to reduced oxygen transport in the blood to the heart (Fig. 27.2).

Q4 When should you begin to investigate and treat anaemia in a patient with CKD?

As the haemoglobin falls below 110 g/l it is appropriate to determine the levels of iron, B12 and folate and replace if required. Because of concerns regarding the potential risks of ESA therapy it is not normally started until the haemoglobin drops below 100 g/l.

> **Box 27.1 Haemoglobin Threshold for Action**
> Hb <110 g/L = Investigate (see following)
> Hb <100 g/L = Start ESA (if needed)
> Hb >115 g/L = Suspend ESA therapy

Q5 How do you determine the likely cause or causes of anaemia in a renal patient?

Iron deficiency is the most common cause. If there is iron deficiency then GI blood loss should be considered and investigated while replacing the iron in an appropriate form. B12 and folate deficiency are less common but will respond to appropriate replacement. If iron, B12 and folate are all normal and if the reticulocyte count is low then ACEI/ARBs should be considered as possible causes of anaemia. Following a full history and examination patients should have an anaemia screen as shown in Fig. 27.3.

M. Findlay, C. Isles, *Clinical Companion in Nephrology*,
DOI 10.1007/978-3-319-14868-7_27, © Springer International Publishing Switzerland 2015

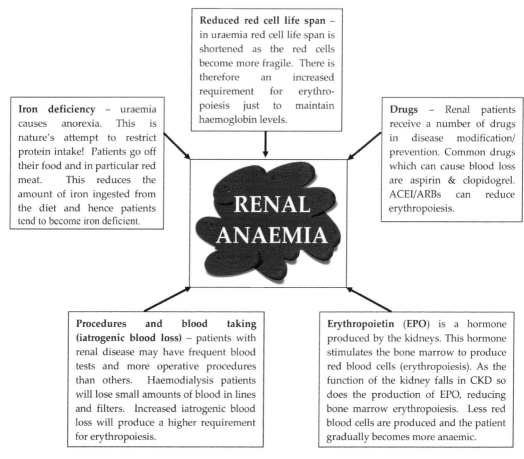

Reduced red cell life span – in uraemia red cell life span is shortened as the red cells become more fragile. There is therefore an increased requirement for erythropoiesis just to maintain haemoglobin levels.

Iron deficiency – uraemia causes anorexia. This is nature's attempt to restrict protein intake! Patients go off their food and in particular red meat. This reduces the amount of iron ingested from the diet and hence patients tend to become iron deficient.

Drugs – Renal patients receive a number of drugs in disease modification/prevention. Common drugs which can cause blood loss are aspirin & clopidogrel. ACEI/ARBs can reduce erythropoiesis.

RENAL ANAEMIA

Procedures and blood taking (iatrogenic blood loss) – patients with renal disease may have frequent blood tests and more operative procedures than others. Haemodialysis patients will lose small amounts of blood in lines and filters. Increased iatrogenic blood loss will produce a higher requirement for erythropoiesis.

Erythropoietin (EPO) is a hormone produced by the kidneys. This hormone stimulates the bone marrow to produce red blood cells (erythropoiesis). As the function of the kidney falls in CKD so does the production of EPO, reducing bone marrow erythropoiesis. Less red blood cells are produced and the patient gradually becomes more anaemic.

Fig. 27.1 Factors influencing renal anaemia

Fig. 27.2 Symptoms of anaemia. The speed of onset of anaemia is clinically very important. A rapid drop = more symptoms and lower Hb = more symptoms. Patients with slowly worsening anaemia often display very few symptoms

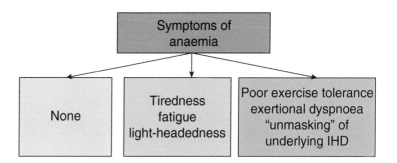

Symptoms of anaemia

None

Tiredness fatigue light-headedness

Poor exercise tolerance exertional dyspnoea "unmasking" of underlying IHD

Q6 What does the serum ferritin tell us and how do we use serum ferritin to make decisions on treatment?

Serum ferritin gives a measure of the body's iron stores. It is also an inflammatory marker which means that it rises when a patient becomes infected e.g. septicaemia or develops some other inflammatory process e.g. rheumatoid arthritis. In other words ferritin is normal or raised when iron stores are acceptable or something in the body is inflamed. Because of this it is not possible to interpret serum ferritin unless you also know the CRP (see below) which is another and perhaps better known inflammatory marker.

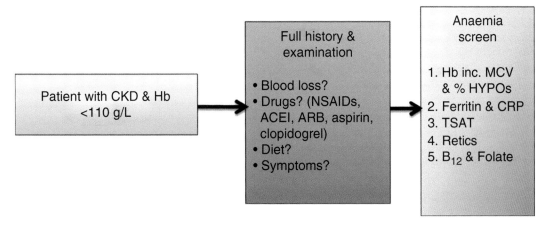

Fig. 27.3 Initial investigation of anaemia in renal disease

Q7 Why is it important to measure CRP when you measure ferritin?

CRP stands for C-reactive protein. The normal level for CRP is less than 3. CRP rises in the presence of infection e.g. septicaemia or other inflammatory processes e.g. rheumatoid arthritis. It is always best to measure CRP when you measure serum ferritin to guide the interpretation of serum ferritin, as follows:

- If serum ferritin is less than 100 µ/L then body iron stores are likely to be low and the patient will respond to iron therapy.
- If the ferritin is greater than 100 µ/L and the CRP is normal, then iron stores are likely to be normal.
- If ferritin is greater than 100 µ/L and the CRP is high then you cannot use serum ferritin to estimate iron stores.

Q8 What is the Transferrin Saturation and how does it help in the management of renal anaemia?

Transferrin saturation or TSAT is the serum iron divided by something called the total iron binding capacity. In patients who are iron deficient the serum iron falls and the total iron binding capacity rises (this is the body's way of holding on to every scrap of iron it can). The problem with this test is the marked diurnal variation in the level of serum iron, which simply means that iron levels can fluctuate quite markedly even during the course of a single day. Nevertheless, a transferrin saturation less than 30 % suggests iron deficiency.

Q9 What further investigations might you undertake in a renal patient who is found to be iron deficient?

The concern for all iron deficient patient over the age of 50 whether they have renal failure or not, is that they might be losing blood from the gastrointestinal tract. It is important to exclude gastric and colon cancer in such patients and necessary to undertake both upper GI endoscopy & colonoscopy. Colonoscopy is the investigation of choice to exclude lower GI bleeding, as it will detect both angiodysplasia and tumours. CT colonography can be used for frail patients to exclude tumours but not angiodysplasia. Both colonscopy and CT colonography are preferable to barium enema.

Causes of Anaemia

You should not assume that all anaemic patients with CKD have renal anaemia – look for reversible/malignant causes elsewhere before treating.

Q10 A haemodialysis patient is found to have a haemoglobin of 100 g/l with evidence of iron deficiency. What is the correct treatment?

Haemodialysis patients have an average iron loss of 50 mg weekly just because of the dialysis procedures. They will require IV iron. Having first undertaken tests to exclude GI blood loss, the correct treatment is to give a loading dose of 1 g intravenous iron. This is best given by using iron saccharate (Venofer) 100 mg (5 ml) IV at each dialysis session for ten doses. See Appendix 12 for more advice on iron therapy.

Q11 When would you use erythropoietin stimulating agents (ESA) such as darbepoietin (Aranesp) to treat anaemia in patients with CKD?

If the patient is still anaemic (Hb <100 g/L) after investigating and treating iron, B12 and folate deficiency and ruling out GI blood loss, then you can assume that the anaemia is because of low EPO levels. ESAs stimulate erythropoiesis in a very similar way to natural erythropoietin. They are given by injection either SC or IV. They comes as pre-filled syringes which means that patients can be taught to self-administer in the same way that people with diabetes give themselves insulin. ESAs are often given weekly in HD patients and fortnightly/monthly in PD or clinic patients. The recommended starting dose for Aranesp in a haemodialysis patient is usually 30 μg weekly. See Appendix 12 for more advice on ESA therapy.

Q12 What are the risks of ESAs?

ESAs are not without risks. They tend to worsen pre-existing hypertension often requiring an increase in anti-hypertensives, and may increase the risk of fistula thrombosis. Fistula thrombosis is thought to be secondary to an increase in the platelet count and an increase in platelet stickiness. Longer term risks to a renal patient taking an ESA whose haemoglobin is consistently greater than 120 g/l are heart attack and strokes, possibly reflecting a prothrombotic effect of the drug. In addition, ESAs should be used with caution in patients with malignancy as they have the potential to increase tumour growth

Q13 Why not simply transfuse a renal patient who has become anaemic?

Transfusion is certainly a quick fix and may well be indicated if a patient is actively bleeding and/or has haemoglobin less than 70 g/l, but in most instances it is better to treat the anaemia with ESA and iron. Transfusion carries three spe-cific risks which are often more significant in renal patients: risks from blood volume, risk of hyperkalaemia and immunological complications. Transfusion should be avoided in all patients who may be transplanted as it may stimulate the production of HLA antibodies and make matching difficult in the future. Transfusion does however have a place in the management of patients with limited life expectancy or a severely unresponsive marrow.

Q14 What if a CKD patient becomes anaemic post operatively?

CKD patients may have a reasonable Hb but in the face of blood loss due to an operation or perhaps a fracture, they are unable to produce enough endogenous erythropoietin to raise their Hb. In this situation they may require ESA for a limited period until their Hb is back to normal. It must also be remembered that they will use more iron during this time and may require temporary iron replacement too.

Q15 A patient on an ESA fails to show the expected rise in haemoglobin. Why might this be?

Patients taking ESAs will fail to respond under the following circumstances:
1. Deficiency of iron, B12 or folate.
2. Marrow failure e.g. myelodysplastic syndrome
3. Intercurrent infection e.g. septicaemia
4. Inflammation e.g. rheumatoid arthritis.
5. Poorly controlled renal bone disease
6. Malignancy e.g. myeloma

The best way to treat ESA resistance is to correct the underlying cause, but if this is not possible e.g. as in myeloma, then it can often be overcome by increasing the dose of ESA. In myeloma, for example, it may be necessary to use up to 200 μg of Aranesp each week (Fig. 27.4).

Q16 What is the reticulocyte count and how does this help in the management of ESA resistance?

Reticulocytes are brand new red cells. The kidneys usually respond to anaemia by producing EPO which stimulates the production of new red cells in a normally functioning bone marrow causing the reticulocyte count in the peripheral

Fig. 27.4 The ESA pathway. Effective erythropoiesis requires iron, B12, folate and erythopoetin. Deficiencies in any of these essential components can result in anaemia. In advanced renal disease, EPO is not produced, necessitating the need for exogenous ESA. As shown, there are certain circumstances where despite adequate stimulation the bone marrow fails to respond

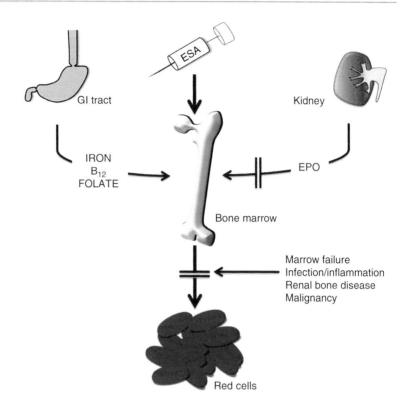

GI tract

ESA

Kidney

IRON
B$_{12}$
FOLATE

EPO

Bone marrow

Marrow failure
Infection/inflammation
Renal bone disease
Malignancy

Red cells

blood to rise. A renal patient with anaemia (say haemoglobin <100 g/l) and a low reticulocyte count (<50) has a marrow that is either not being stimulated or not working. This either means lack of EPO or that their marrow has been suppressed by marrow failure, infection, inflammation, poorly controlled renal bone disease or malignancy. Some drugs, particularly ACEIs and mycophenolate, may also reduce the marrow response to ESA causing a low reticulocyte anaemia. If the reticulocyte count is normal or high (>50), then the bone marrow response is good and you should look instead for sources of blood loss.

27.1 Objectives: Renal Anaemia

After reading this chapter, you should be able to answer the following:

Q1 What is haemoglobin and what are the normal levels?

Q2 Why do patients with CKD (chronic kidney disease) become anaemic?

Q3 What are the symptoms of anaemia?

Q4 When should you begin to investigate and treat anaemia in a patient with CKD?

Q5 How do you determine the likely cause or causes of anaemia in a renal patient?

Q6 What does the serum ferritin tell us and how do we use serum ferritin to make decisions on treatment?

Q7 Why is it important to measure CRP when you measure ferritin?

Q8 What is the Transferrin Saturation and how does it help in the management of renal anaemia?

Q9 What further investigations might you undertake in a renal patient who is found to be iron deficient?

Q10 A haemodialysis patient is found to have a haemoglobin of 100 g/l with evidence of

Q2 Why do patients with CKD develop disorders of mineral metabolism?

Two things happen when GFR falls below 30 ml/min. Serum phosphate rises – simply because the kidneys cannot excrete it – and serum calcium begins to fall because the failing kidney cannot activate vitamin D. Vitamin D is normally responsible for increasing the absorption of calcium from the gut. Failure to activate vitamin D therefore leads to hypocalcaemia. Hyperphosphataemia also leads to hypocalcaemia, at least partly because of failure to activate vitamin D (Fig. 28.2).

Q3 What do you understand by the term secondary hyperparathyroidism?

Secondary hyperparathyroidism occurs when the parathyroid gland is stimulated to secrete PTH by low serum calcium and high serum phosphate. PTH does its best to correct hyperphosphataemia by reducing phosphate reabsorption in the kidney. Its main action, however, is to raise serum calcium. It does this in three ways:

1. By direct action on the kidney increasing calcium reabsorption.
2. Indirectly, by activating vitamin D which then increases absorption of calcium from the gut.
3. By stimulating the osteoclasts in bone. Osteoclasts break down bone releasing calcium into the blood stream.

The ability of the failing kidney to regulate calcium and phosphate reabsorption and to activate vitamin D may then become exhausted, leaving osteoclastic reabsorption of bone as the only way left of normalising serum calcium (Fig. 28.3). As a consequence of increased osteoclastic activity, there is secondary stimulation of new bone formation by osteoblasts, the activity of which is reflected by the level of the enzyme alkaline phosphatase in the blood stream. When all these features are present, secondary hyperparathyroidism is characterised by a low (may sometimes be normal) serum calcium, high serum phosphate, high serum PTH±high serum alkaline phosphatase.

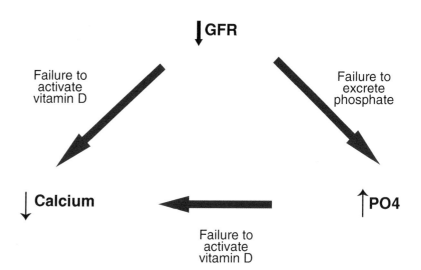

Fig. 28.2 Mechanism through which renal failure causes hypocalcaemia and hyperphosphataemia

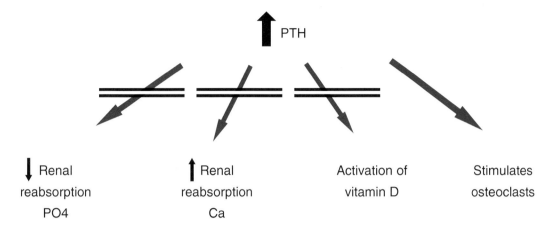

Fig. 28.3 Actions of PTH in renal disease

Q4   What are the clinical features of secondary hyperparathyroidism?

The condition may be completely asymptomatic but may also be characterised by bone pain or fractures. The risk of fracture is increased by the other forms of bone disease, particularly osteoporosis.

Q5   Why do renal patients sometimes develop osteomalacia?

Osteomalacia means failure to mineralise bone adequately and in renal osteomalacia accumulation of aluminium may be responsible. Historically renal osteomalacia occurred in haemodialysis patients before we began removing aluminium from the dialysis water by reverse osmosis. Nowadays renal osteomalacia is seen occasionally in patients who are taking aluminium as a phosphate binder, which is one of the reasons why Alucaps are used less than before.

Q6   Why does soft tissue calcification occur?

Soft tissue calcification, also known as metastatic calcification, describes the deposition of calcium and phosphate in soft tissue such as muscles, joints and arteries. This occurs in all kidney patients but particularly in those in whom the calcium phosphate product (serum calcium × serum phosphate) exceeds 4.5 mmol/L. Arterial calcification may contribute to the high rates of vascular disease seen in renal patients, and is one of the reasons for the move away from calcium containing phosphate binders such as Calcichew and Phosex.

> **Calcium & Phosphate Product = Serum Calcium × Serum Phosphate**.
> If this exceeds 4.5, there is significant risk of soft tissue or "metastatic" calcification. Reducing levels of phosphate by binders while maintaining a normal serum calcium is key to treatment.

A flow chart summarising the pathogenesis of secondary hyperparathyroidism, osteomalacia and soft tissue calcification is shown overleaf (Fig. 28.4).

Q7   What is adynamic bone disease?

In health, bone is continuously broken down & rebuilt. Adynamic bone disease is a condition in which this process of "turn-over" is absent or depressed. Uraemic patients develop skeletal resistance to PTH so even a normal PTH level may represent reduced bone turnover. A low serum level of parathyroid hormone may also be a consequence of over-suppression of PTH by alfacalcidol. Patients whose bones are not constantly being remodelled are at greater risk of fracture.

Fig. 28.4 Pathogenesis of renal bone disease

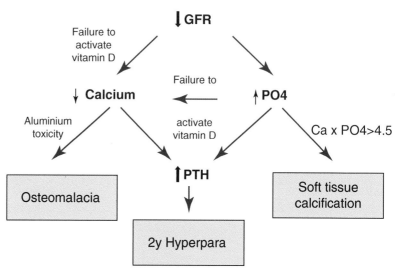

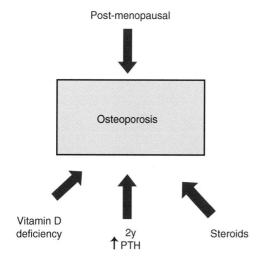

Fig. 28.5 Mechanisms by which renal disease predisposes to osteoporosis

Q8   Why do renal patients develop osteoporosis?

The fifth main disorder of mineral metabolism is osteoporosis, which literally means thin bones. This is an important cause of fracture in renal patients. Renal patients are prone to all the usual causes of osteoporosis eg post-menopausal osteoporosis and have other reasons for developing thin bones which include immobility, vitamin D deficiency, secondary hyperparathyroidism and the use of steroids, particularly after transplantation or the treatment of certain glomerulopathies (Fig. 28.5).

Q9   What should you measure and when?

As general rule patients do not develop disorders of mineral metabolism until they reach CKD stage 4 or 5. When they do so you should check serum calcium, phosphate, PTH and 25(OH)D in order to obtain a set of baseline measurements. The subsequent frequency of testing will be determined by the results and clinical circumstances.

Q10   What are the biochemical targets for controlling secondary hyperparathyroidism?

There are three. The first is to keep the serum phosphate between 0.9 and 1.5 mmol/l (1.1–1.7 mmol/L in dialysis patients). The second is to maintain serum calcium within the normal range for your hospital. The third target is to maintain the serum PTH at an acceptable level. Unfortunately, there is no optimal PTH level known for patients with CKD not on dialysis and so treatment with active vitamin D is recommended when modifiable factors (hypocalcaemia, hyperphosphataemia and hypovitaminosis D) have been corrected. In the dialysis population it is recommenced to maintain PTH between 2 and 9 times the upper limit of normal (ULN) for your laboratory range (e.g. if a laboratory's normal range is 1.6–6.9 pmol/l, then the target range for serum PTH in patients with renal bone disease is 14–63 pmol/l). The aim is to avoid hypercalcaemia in order to reduce the risk of arterial calcification and also to avoid suppressing PTH to <14 pmol/l to reduce the risk of adynamic bone disease.

Box 28.1 Bone targets for CKD (and for dialysis in brackets)

PO$_4$	0.9–1.5 mmol/L (1.1–1.7 mmol/L)
Calcium	Normal range for hospital (same)
PTH	Treat if progressive rise (maintain at 2–9× ULN)

Q11 What can be done to treat secondary hyperparathyroidism?

You can think of this under the following headings:

Box 28.2 Treatment Strategies for Renal Bone Disease

1. **Measures that lower serum phosphate**
   (a) Dietary restriction of phosphate.
   (b) Elimination of phosphate by dialysis
   (c) Oral phosphate binders.
2. **Measures that increase serum calcium**
   (a) By lowering PO$_4$ (as above)
   (b) By alfacalcidol, the active metabolite of vitamin D.
3. **Keeping PTH within recommended range**
   (a) By alfacalcidol (as above)
   (b) By cinacalcet (Mimpara), a drug which restores the sensitivity of the parathyroid gland to stimulation by calcium.
   (c) Parathyroidectomy.

The reality is that for most patients this will mean using a combination of phosphate binders and alfacalcidol. Dietary phosphate restriction is difficult, particularly as phosphate is found in dairy products. Changing to a bigger dialyser does not usually help because phosphate is primarily intracellular and only cleared poorly by 12 h dialysis per week. The indications for Cinacalcet and parathyroidectomy are given below.

Q12 Discuss the use of phosphate binders in secondary hyperparathyroidism

Such drugs are introduced when the serum phosphate rises and is consistently above 1.5 mmol/l (CKD patients) or 1.7 mmol/L (on dialysis). There are four types of phosphate binder each with their own advantages and limitations, as follows:

Box 28.3 Phosphate Binders

1. Calcium acetate (Phosex) or carbonate (Calcichew)	Calcium containing PO$_4$ binders
2. Aluminium hydroxide (Alucaps)	Aluminium containing PO$_4$ binder
3. Sevelemar hydrochloride (Renagel) or carbonate (Renvela)	Non-calcium, non-aluminium PO$_4$ binders
4. Lanthanum (Fosrenol)	Another non-calcium, non-aluminium, PO$_4$ binder

---

All of these drugs work by binding phosphate in the diet. Calcium binders, aluminium hydroxide and sevelemar must all be taken just before eating in order to be effective. The exception to this rule is lanthanum which should be given towards end of the meal or immediately after food otherwise the patient will vomit. A common mistake made by non-renal medical staff is to prescribe these drugs three times daily at 6 am, 2 pm and 10 pm, rather than at meal times. Giving phosphate binders between meals is pointless. In severe 2y and 3y hyperparathyroidism phosphate binders are less effective because the high serum phosphate is derived from bone not diet. For more details on how to use phosphate binders see Appendix 13.

Phosphate Binders

PO$_4$ binders bind dietary phosphate. Therefore, they must be given WITH FOOD to be effective; either before (Phosex, Calcichew, Alucaps, Sevelemar) or after (Lanthanum) meals.

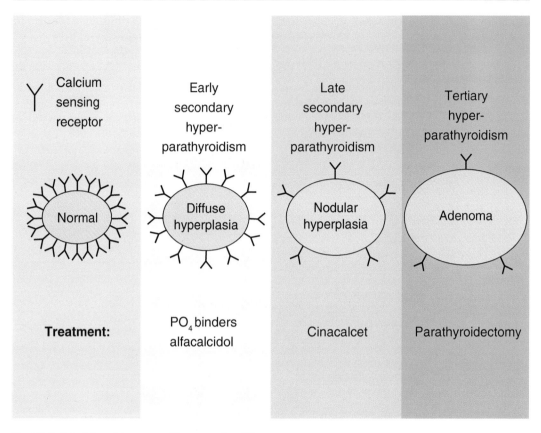

Fig. 28.6 Principles of the stages of hyperparathyroidism

Q13   How does the action of calcium carbonate differ from that of calcium resonium?

Medical students frequently confuse the mechanism of action of these two drugs. Calcium carbonate binds the phosphate in food preventing its absorption from the gut. Calcium resonium is a resin used in the management of some patients with hyperkalaemia. The resin sits in the small intestine and exchanges potassium for hydrogen across the bowel wall. It does not require to be taken with food because it does not bind dietary potassium.

Q14   What do you understand by the term tertiary hyperparathyroidism?

When the PTH gland has been over-stimulated for a long time the gland enlarges and begins to lose its calcium sensing receptors. This is associated with diffuse hyperplasia then nodular hyperplasia and finally the formation of one or more parathyroid adenomas. By the time a parathyroid adenoma has developed there are so few calcium sensing receptors that serum PTH can no longer be suppressed by high serum calcium. This condition is called tertiary hyperparathyroidism. Treatment is by parathyroidectomy to remove the autonomously functioning gland or glands (Fig. 28.6).

Q15   What are the indications for using cinacalcet (Mimpara)?

Cinacalcet acts on whatever calcium sensing receptors remain in the parathyroid gland to restore their sensitivity to calcium. It is useful in patients with severe or late secondary hyperparathyroidism where serum phosphate is uncontrolled and PTH is greater than 80 pmol/l. If successful then serum calcium, phosphate and PTH will all fall, enabling alfacalcidol to be restarted. Calcium, phosphate and PTH should be checked weekly when introducing cinacalcet or adjusting the dose. The dose range is 30–180 mg daily. Cinacalcet is expensive and may best be regarded as a parathyroidectomy sparing treatment.

Q16 What are the indications for parathyroidectomy?

Parathyroidectomy in end stage renal disease is performed primarily in symptomatic patients with markedly elevated and non-suppressible serum PTH values. Patients will therefore generally have serum PTH greater than 80 pmol/l with one or more of the following:
- Severe hypercalcaemia.
- Pruritis that does not respond to medical therapy or dialysis.
- Progressive soft tissue calcification.
- Calciphylaxis – a rare and serious disorder characterised by vascular calcification in arterioles that leads to ischaemia and subcutaneous necrosis.
- Otherwise unexplained symptomatic myopathy.

Hypocalcaemia is extremely common post op because calcium is sucked from the blood back into the bones when it is no longer under the influence of PTH (so called hungry bone syndrome). The management of hungry bone syndrome is given in Appendix 14.

Q17 How do you treat osteoporosis in patients with CKD?

The indications for oral bisphosphonates for the prevention and treatment of osteoporosis in CKD3 are the same as for people who do not have CKD. None of the guidelines give advice for patients whose eGFR is lower than this. We and others have used risedronate at a reduced dose of 5 mg once weekly for CKD 4/5 including dialysis patients, though we recognise that this is an unlicensed indication. We avoid bisphosphonates altogether if serum PTH is low as there is a theoretical risk they might provoke or worsen adynamic bone disease.

Q18 How do you treat vitamin D deficiency in patients with CKD?

The important point to note here is that treatment of renal bone disease by alfacalcidol in patients with CKD 4/5 does not correct vitamin D deficiency if that is also present. It is logical therefore to correct vitamin D deficiency first by oral cholecalciferol and then only prescribe alfacalcidol if symptoms or biochemical evidence of secondary hyperparathyroidism persists

28.1 Objectives: Mineral Metabolism

After reading this chapter, you should be able to answer the following:

Q1 List the disorders of mineral metabolism that may occur in chronic kidney disease

Q2 Why do patients with CKD develop disorders of mineral metabolism?

Q3 What do you understand by the term secondary hyperparathyroidism?

Q4 What are the clinical features of secondary hyperparathyroidism?

Q5 Why do renal patients sometimes develop osteomalacia?

Q6 Why does soft tissue calcification occur?

Q7 What is adynamic bone disease?

Q8 Why do renal patients develop osteoporosis?

Q9 What should you measure and when?

Q10 What are the biochemical targets for controlling secondary hyperparathyroidism?

Q11 What can be done to treat secondary hyperparathyroidism?

Q12 Discuss the use of phosphate binders in secondary hyperparathyroidism?

Q13 How does the action of calcium carbonate differ from that of calcium resonium?

Q14 What do you understand by the term tertiary hyperparathyroidism?

Q15 What are the indications for using Cinacalcet (Mimpara)?

Q16 What are the indications for parathyroidectomy?

Q17 How do you treat osteoporosis in patients with CKD?

Q18 How do you treat vitamin D deficiency in patients with CKD?

Further Reading

1. Kidney Disease: Improving Global Outcomes (KDIGO) CKD–MBD Work Group. KDIGO clinical practice guideline for the diagnosis, evaluation, prevention, and treatment of chronic kidney disease–mineral and bone disorder (CKD–MBD). Kidney Int Suppl. 2009;76 Suppl 113:S1–130.
2. Steddon S, Sharples E. Clinical Practice Guideline. CKD mineral and bone disorders (CKD-MBD). UK Renal Association, 2013. www.renal.org/guideline/modules/ckd-mineral-and-bone-disorders.

Q1 Why might patients with kidney disease need dietary advice?

Malnutrition is common, affecting up to 50 % of patients with renal disease. It has an adverse impact on mortality rates. Patients with CKD stages 4 or 5 often present with potassium and phosphate electrolyte imbalance which will require dietetic management. Patients on dialysis usually produce little or no urine and frequently require education in relation to fluid and sodium restriction to prevent fluid overload.

Q2 When should a renal patient be referred to a renal dietitian?

When CKD reaches stage 4 and 5. Other than advice to reduce sodium intake, most patients with CKD stage 3 do not require the expertise of a specialist renal dietician.

Q3 What sort of dietary advice is a renal patient likely to require?

This will vary considerably both between and within patients as they move from pre-dialysis through peritoneal dialysis and haemodialysis to transplantation. It is likely however that specific dietary advice will be required in one or more of the following areas of nutritional intake:

> **Box 29.1 Areas for Dietary Discussion**
> Protein
> Energy
> Potassium
> Phosphate
> Fluid
> Sodium

Q4 What advice might you give a renal patient with CKD 4–5 regarding their protein intake?

Debate continues as to the optimal level of protein intake in stages 4–5. High protein diets should be avoided as they increase hyperfiltration, worsen proteinuria and speed the decline of renal function. There was once a vogue for low protein diets as a means of preventing uraemic symptoms in the run up to dialysis but this advice has long been abandoned as it only led to malnutrition. Currently, for patients not on dialysis a minimum daily protein of 0.75 g/kg ideal body weight is recommended.

Q5 What advice might you give a renal patient with CKD 4–5 regarding their energy intake?

Energy expenditure is similar to that of healthy individuals. An intake of 35 kcal/kg/day should

M. Findlay, C. Isles, *Clinical Companion in Nephrology*,
DOI 10.1007/978-3-319-14868-7_29, © Springer International Publishing Switzerland 2015

be adequate for most patients. It is important to ensure an adequate energy intake in order to prevent negative nitrogen balance and weight loss. This is particularly likely to occur in patients whose appetites are poor and in those who have other comorbidities such as cardiac and respiratory disease.

Q6 What advice might you give a renal patient with CKD 4–5 regarding their potassium intake?

Hyperkalaemia becomes increasingly common as GFR falls. Average daily potassium intake in the UK is 50–100 mmol. Higher intakes than this may lead to hyperkalaemia in patients with CKD 4–5 particularly if they also happen to be taking ACEIs or ARBs for their proteinuria or hypertension. The level of potassium restriction should be individualised according to dietary intake, blood levels and medical treatment. Non-essential foods should be limited or avoided first, e.g. coffee and chocolate. Other high potassium foods such as fruit, vegetables, potatoes, meat and milk are important components of the diet and should not be restricted unnecessarily. Potassium restriction is likely to be necessary when serum K exceeds 5.5 mmol/l. Advice on how to do this is given in Appendix 9.

Q7 What advice might you give a renal patient with CKD 4–5 regarding their phosphate intake?

Hyperphosphataemia >1.5 mmol/l is an important cause of secondary hyperparathyroidism. Phosphate also binds with calcium in the blood to cause itchy skin and soft tissue calcification. A low phosphate diet (see Appendix 10) is then recommended, although phosphate binders are also often required (for more information on phosphate binders see Chap. 28). Current UK guidelines recommend that serum phosphate be maintained between 0.9 and 1.5 mmol/L for CKD stages 4 and 5 who are not on dialysis.

Q8 What advice might you give a renal patient with CKD 4–5 regarding their fluid intake?

Most people drink 1–2 litres/day and do not need to restrict fluid intake until their kidney failure is very advanced (CKD 5) and only then if they are oedematous. Patients who find fluid restriction difficult or impossible because they are thirsty should cut down on salt. Fluid restriction becomes a much bigger issue on dialysis (see Q10).

Q9 What advice might you give a renal patient with CKD 4–5 regarding their sodium intake?

Average sodium intake in the UK is around 150–200 mmol (equivalent to 9–12 g of salt) which is considerably more than required physiologically. High sodium intake contributes to hypertension and to fluid retention both of which are common in renal patients. Dietitians will recommend adding a pinch of salt to cooking, avoiding processed foods if possible and not adding salt at table in an attempt to reduce sodium intake to around 100 mmol per day. Patients accustomed to a high salt diet should be warned that their food may lose its taste for a few weeks until their taste buds adjust to a lower salt intake. They should also be advised to avoid salt substitutes such as Lo-Salt which contain large amounts of potassium.

Q10 In what way would your nutritional advice differ for patients who are already on dialysis?

Higher protein intakes of 1.2 g/kg ideal body weight are recommended both for HD and PD patients because of protein losses in dialysis fluids. Recommended energy requirements are 35 kcal/kg/day, reflecting their catabolic state. The need for dietary potassium and phosphate restriction, and for phosphate binders, should be determined by serum levels, as for pre-dialysis patients. Dialysis will clear potassium and phosphate from the blood stream but levels will rebound because both cations are predominantly intracellular. Patients usually find fluid and salt restriction the most challenging of all the advice they receive. The need to restrict will depend to a great extent on the amount of urine they continue to pass. It is advised the HD patients limit their interdialytic weight gain to a maximum of 2 kg whilst often accepted that PD patients who ultra-filtrate poorly will be chronically overloaded.

29.1   Nutrition in Renal Disease

Q1   **Why might patients with kidney disease need dietary advice?**

Q2   **When should a renal patient be referred to a renal dietitian?**

Q3   **What sort of dietary advice is a renal patient likely to require?**

Q4   **What advice might you give a renal patient with CKD 4–5 regarding their protein intake?**

Q5   **What advice might you give a renal patient with CKD 4–5 regarding their energy intake?**

Q6   **What advice might you give a renal patient with CKD 4–5 regarding their potassium intake?**

Q7   **What advice might you give a renal patient with CKD 4–5 regarding their phosphate intake?**

Q8   **What advice might you give a renal patient with CKD 4–5 regarding their fluid intake?**

Q9   **What advice might you give a renal patient with CKD 4–5 regarding their sodium intake?**

Q10 **In what way would your nutritional advice differ for patients who are already on dialysis?**

Gout and the Kidney

Q1 What is gout?

Gout is the most common form of inflammatory arthritis affecting 1.5 % of the UK population. Various clinical presentations exist with an underlying common pathophysiology of urate crystal deposition within tissues causing inflammation and tissue damage. The key risk factor is hyperuricaemia.

Q2 Why are kidney patients at risk?

A raised serum urate is common in chronic kidney disease, predominantly from a combination of impaired clearance and diuretic use. Although many patients with hyperuricaemia remain asymptomatic, some will present with an acute attack of gout. Less commonly, acute kidney injury due to uric acid nephropathy may be seen as part of the acute tumour lysis syndrome in patients undergoing chemotherapy or radiation therapy for the treatment of malignancies with rapid cell turnover, such as leukemia and lymphoma.

Q3 How would you diagnose an acute attack of gout in a renal patient?

In much the same way as you would diagnose gout in a patient who does not have renal disease, namely with pain, inflammation and often immobility of a single joint. Eighty percent of presentations involve the lower limb. Important clues to the diagnosis are involvement of the first MTP joint and the presence of gouty tophi, but gout should be considered in a differential diagnosis of any kidney patient with monoarthritis. The

demonstration of negatively birefringent uric acid crystals in joint fluid is pathognomonic for acute gout though it is frequently not possible to obtain a sample of joint fluid, for example if the first MTP joint is the only joint involved.

Q4 What other causes are there of a hot swollen joint in a patient with CKD?

The most important is probably septic arthritis. Leucocytosis and fever may be present in both. The only certain way to distinguish septic arthritis from acute gout is by aspiration and culture of joint fluid. The distinction is critical because the treatment of gout is with anti-inflammatory drugs and the treatment of septic arthritis is with a prolonged course of antibiotic. Pseudogout, which often presents as a hot swollen knee in elderly with OA, is another important differential. Patients with pseudogout have chondrocalcinosis on x-ray & rhomboid crystals of calcium pyrophosphate in synovial fluid.

Q5 How useful is the serum uric acid in the treatment and prevention of gout?

Serum uric acid is not helpful in diagnosis but is an important target for prevention. Not every patient with hyperuricaemia will develop gout and serum uric acid may fall during an acute attack, becoming falsely negative. Serum uric acid is an important target for prevention of gout with drugs that inhibit its production, the doses of which should be increased until the serum uric acid falls below 0.30 mmol/l, if tolerated.

M. Findlay, C. Isles, *Clinical Companion in Nephrology*,
DOI 10.1007/978-3-319-14868-7_30, © Springer International Publishing Switzerland 2015

Q6 How would you treat an acute attack of gout in a patient without CKD?

Treat as soon as possible with NSAIDs, colchicine or steroids. NSAIDs should be given in full doses. There is no evidence to suggest that any one NSAID is better than any other. The starting dose of colchicine for acute gout in patients with normal renal function is 1 mg stat then 0.5 mg tds until the attack resolves or gastrointestinal side effects develop. Prednisolone 40 mg once daily for 5–10 days is an effective alternative if NSAIDs or colchicine are contraindicated or poorly tolerated. Allopurinol should not be started during an acute attack but in patients already established on allopurinol, it should be continued and the acute attack treated conventionally. Opiate analgesics can be used as adjuncts. Rest, cold packs and splintage can be helpful.

Q7 How does management of the acute attack differ in a patient with CKD?

The options are the same but NSAIDs and colchicine are relatively contraindicated. NSAIDs may cause a reversible decline in renal function. This might be acceptable if given for a few days to patients whose renal function is only mildly impaired but generally they are best avoided. The impact on renal function is less relevant on regular dialysis although the use of NSAIDs is often then limited by hyperkalaemia and GI upset. Colchicine is cleared by the kidney. Some patients can abort an acute attack of gout by taking 0.5–1 mg at the very first twinge but higher doses are not recommended when GFR <60 ml/min and for this reason a short course of prednisolone may be the best option.

Q8 What do you need to know about colchicine?

Colchicine is a natural product derived from Colchicum autumnale (aka the autumn crocus), approved for use both as monotherapy for the treatment of acute gout and for the prevention of gout flares. It is frequently given for up to 6 months to prevent acute attacks during initiation of anti-hyperuricaemic therapy. Colchicine is of limited value when acute gout occurs with CKD for reasons already discussed though it can be used prophylactically provided the dose is adjusted as GFR falls (Box 30.1). Colchicine has three important side effects, all of which are more common in CKD. These are vomiting, diarrhoea and neutropenia. Vomiting and diarrhoea are dose related while neutropenia is most likely to occur if colchicine is given with CYP3A4 inhibitors such as clarithromycin.

Box 30.1 Colchicine Prophylaxis in CKD

eGFR	Dose and frequency
≥60 ml/min	0.5 mg once or twice daily
30–59 ml/min	0.5 mg once daily or every other day
<30 ml/min	0.5 mg every 2–3 days

Q9 Should all patients with gout be offered prophylactic therapy with allopurinol?

The British Society for Rheumatology recommend drug prophylaxis for patients with gout and renal insufficiency (eGFR <60 ml/min) in addition to the following groups: those with uncomplicated gout if second or further attacks within 1 year; with visible gouty tophi; with uric acid stones; and patients who need to continue to take diuretics

Q10 What do you need to know about allopurinol?

Allopurinol is a purine based xanthine oxidase inhibitor that inhibits production of uric acid. It is first line drug therapy for prevention of recurrent gout but has no place in management of acute gout and may even trigger an acute attack if given alone so is usually co-prescribed with colchicine. The starting dose is 100–300 mg daily in patients with normal renal function. Lower starting doses are recommended in patients with CKD – see Box 30.2. Allopurinol should be increased by 50–100 mg daily every 2–3 weeks if necessary and if tolerated in order to achieve serum uric acid <0.30 mmol/l. Its most important side effect is a skin rash that may vary in severity from mild and remitting with reduction in dose, to severe and life threatening including toxic epidermal necrolysis and Stevens-Johnson syndrome. It also has an important drug interaction with azathioprine that can lead to life threatening neutropenia. Under these circumstances the options are to reduce dose of azathioprine by 75 % or switch to mycophenolate which does not interact with allopurinol.

Box 30.2 Allopurinol Prophylaxis in CKD

eGFR	Initial dose	Dose increment
≥60 ml/min	100–300 mg daily	100 mg every 2–3 weeks
30–59 ml/min	100 mg daily	50–100 mg every 2–3 weeks
<30 ml/min	50 mg daily	50 mg every 2–3 weeks

Q11 What if allopurinol is poorly tolerated or ineffective?

Febuxostat is a recently developed non purine based xanthine oxidase inhibitor that is metabolised by the liver. The dose range is 40–80 mg daily. No dose adjustment is necessary in patients with mild to moderate renal impairment (GFR 30–60 ml/min). Caution is advised at lower GFR levels. Coprescription of febuxostat and azathioprine carries the same risk of neutropenia as allopurinol and azathioprine. Other drugs that can be used to lower uric acid levels include the uricosuric agents probenecid, sulfinpyrazone and losartan though they are seldom effective when GFR <60 ml/min.

Q12 What lifestyle measures are recommended for patients with gout?

Gout has traditionally been regarded as a disorder of the privileged and wealthy and though the stereotype is perhaps a little inaccurate nowadays lifestyle measures have a definite role to play in management. These are to aim for ideal body weight; encourage moderate physical exercise; restrict alcohol intake <21 units for men or <14 units for women, avoid beer and port, with at least 3 alcohol free days each week; drink at least 2 litres of fluid per day; restrict purine intake (Box 30.3). The patient.co.uk website has a useful gout diet sheet which can be printed off and given to patients at clinics.

Box 30.3 High Purine Foods

Meat sources	Liver, heart, kidney, sweetbreads, ox, game (e.g., venison, rabbit), meat extracts (e.g., stock cubes/gravies)
Fish sources	Anchovies, crab, fish roes, herring, mackerel, trout, sardines, shrimps, sprats, whitebait
Other sources	Yeast and extracts, beer, asparagus, cauliflower, mushrooms, beans and peas, spinach

30.1 Objectives: Gout and the Kidney

After reading this chapter, you should be able to answer the following:

Q1 What is gout?

Q2 Why are kidney patients at risk?

Q3 How would you diagnose an acute attack of gout in a renal patient?

Q4 What other causes are there of a hot swollen joint in a patient with CKD?

Q5 How useful is the serum uric acid in the treatment and prevention of gout?

Q6 How would you treat an acute attack of gout in a patient without CKD?

Q7 How does management of the acute attack differ in a patient with CKD?

Q8 What do you need to know about colchicine?

Q9   Should all patients with gout be offered prophylactic therapy with allopurinol?

Q10 What do you need to know about allopurinol?

Q11 What if allopurinol is poorly tolerated or ineffective?

Q12 What lifestyle measures are recommended for patients with gout?

Further Reading

1. Jordan KM, et al. British Society for Rheumatology and British Health Professionals in Rheumatology Guideline for the Management of Gout. Rheumatology. 2007;46(8):1372–74. Accessed online 30/09/2014 via http://www.rheumatology.org.uk/includes/documents/cm_docs/2009/m/management_of_gout.pdf.
2. Khanna D, et al. 2012 American College of Rheumatology Guidelines for Management of Gout. Parts 1 and 2. Arthritis Care Res. 2012;62(10):1431–6; 1447–61.

Q1 How does urinary tract infection present clinically?

Acute cystitis is the most common presentation. Elderly patients frequently present with asymptomatic bacteriuria. Acute pyelonephritis is suggested by the triad of fever with loin pain and loin tenderness. Acute prostatitis may cause pain or achiness in the abdomen above the pubic bone, in the lower back, in the perineum or testicles, in addition to symptoms of UTI. Urinary tract infection is an important cause of gram negative septicaemia in patients who are admitted to hospital. The full spectrum of presentations of urinary tract infection is shown the Box 31.1.

> **Box 31.1 Presentations of Urinary Tract Infection**
> - Acute cystitis
> - Asymptomatic bacteriuria
> - Acute pyelonephritis.
> - Acute prostatitis.
> - Gram negative septicaemia.

Q2 Describe the typical clinical features of cystitis

These are one or more of sudden onset of frequency of micturition with urgency, a burning pain in the urethra when passing urine (dysuria), an intense desire to pass more urine after micturition (strangury), cloudy urine with an unpleasant smell, visible or non visible haematuria.

Somewhat less typically cystitis may present with collapse, delirium, urinary retention, abdominal pain and agitation, particularly in the elderly.

Q3 What other causes of lower urinary tract symptoms do you know?

In females, it is probably best to consider these as being with or without vaginal discharge. Those with vaginal discharge include thrush, sexually transmitted disease, malignancy, physical irritation from IUDs and diaphragms and chemical irritation from latex condoms (latex free condoms are available). Some women present with frequency and dysuria but have no bacteria in their urine and no vaginal discharge, the so-called "urethral syndrome". Possible explanations include bacteria that are difficult to culture, a chemical irritation to toiletries, symptoms relating to sexual intercourse and atrophic vaginitis. In men, by far the most common presentation in the absence of infection is that of prostatism presenting with frequency of urination, terminal dribbling, nocturia and hesitancy.

Q4 What other diagnoses should you consider in patients with loin pain?

An obstructing renal stone is the obvious answer. Pain will usually radiate from loin to groin and be associated with visible or non-visible haematuria. In all women of child bearing age with loin pain consider possibility of ectopic pregnancy and request a pregnancy test.

M. Findlay, C. Isles, *Clinical Companion in Nephrology*,
DOI 10.1007/978-3-319-14868-7_31, © Springer International Publishing Switzerland 2015

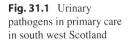 **Fig. 31.1** Urinary
pathogens in primary care
in south west Scotland

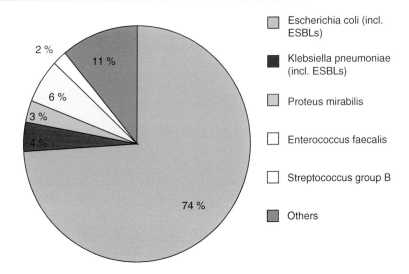

In patients over 55 years of age with loin pain but no other symptoms of UTI consider acute abdominal aortic aneurysm and ask for an urgent surgical opinion.

Q5   Which bacteria are most likely to cause UTI?

E.coli derived from the gastrointestinal tract accounts for around 75 % of all infections. Other bacteria commonly causing community acquired UTI include klebsiella, proteus, enterococcus, streptococcus group B (Fig. 31.1). Proteus infections occur more commonly following instrumentation because they demonstrate an ability to swarm and cover surfaces. A greater variety of organisms and mixed infections occur in patients with catheters or stents and in those who are immunocompromised. Most infections ascend from the perineum to the bladder where they cause acute cystitis. Some then ascend further to the kidney causing acute pyelonephritis.

Q6   Give five important predisposing factors to UTI.

Sexual intercourse may facilitate the transfer of bacteria from the perineum into the bladder. Foreign bodies such as a urethral catheter or ureteric stent are frequently associated with urinary tract infections. Atrophic vaginitis in postmenopausal women and poorly controlled diabe-

tes can lead to loss of host defences. Any cause of urinary retention will allow urine, which is an excellent culture medium for bacteria, to stagnate in the bladder. Vesico-ureteric reflux is an important cause of ascending UTI in childhood. Failing to drink or void when busy on-call is common in conscientious female junior doctors (so called on-call cystitis). Risk factors for UTI are summarised in the box below.

Box 31.2 Risk Factors for Urinary Tract Infections
- Sexual intercourse
- Foreign bodies such as a urethral catheter or ureteric stent
- Loss of host defences such as atrophic vaginitis or poorly controlled diabetes
- Any cause of urinary retention.
- Vesico-ureteric reflux

Q7   What is the role of the urine dipstick test in diagnosing urosepsis?

Urine dipstick tests detect leukocyte esterase and nitrites as surrogates for an elevated urinary white cell count and gram negative bacteriuria respectively. These tests are sensitive but not specific for urosepsis meaning that a negative result makes a urinary infection very unlikely but that a positive result does not confirm. The urine dip is therefore a rule out test.

Q8 Is it always necessary to culture urine before starting antibiotics for suspected UTI?

This depends on the circumstances. Urine culture is not necessary and not recommended by SIGN in an otherwise healthy woman presenting for the first time with acute cystitis, provided that the urine dipstick is positive for nitrites and leucocytes. The absence of both makes UTI extremely unlikely. All other patients i.e. those with recurrent infection, men, the elderly, the immunocompromised should have urine sent for culture before starting antibiotic (though it is not necessary to wait for the result of that culture before prescribing an antibiotic if the presentation is suggestive).

Q9 What is the correct way to obtain a mid-stream specimen of urine (MSU)?

This can be a somewhat delicate and sensitive matter to describe to a patient. Women should wipe themselves from front to back with a saline soaked swab then hold their labia apart before starting to pass urine. They should then pass a sterile aluminium foil bowl in and out of the middle of the stream of urine. This urine should be tipped into a tube containing boric acid (not an universal container) and sent to the lab for gram stain, white cell count, red cell count and culture. The procedure is the same for men except that they must pull back their foreskin, if they have one, and wipe the glans with a saline soaked swab.

Q10 What if a patient who has been admitted to hospital with suspected UTI can't pass urine?

This is a common scenario. Too often patients admitted to hospital with suspected UTI have antibiotics prescribed before urine is sent for culture, thereby making it impossible to know whether the urinary tract was responsible for the sepsis/presumed sepsis. It is therefore essential to dip a specimen of urine and send this for culture before starting antibiotics. Blood cultures are also mandatory in sick patients who may well be septicaemic. Three scenarios for obtaining a urine specimen are given in the box.

> **Box 31.3 Scenarios for Obtaining Urine Specimen**
> - If a patient is not critically ill then ask the nurses to obtain a sample of urine and start antibiotic after the sample has been sent.
> - If a patient is critically ill then they will likely need a urinary catheter to monitor their urine output, which should allow you to obtain a specimen of urine before starting antibiotic.
> - In patients who are not critically ill in whom a urine sample is essential but for a variety of reasons difficult to collect, an in/out catheter sample of urine should be obtained.

Q11 Which antibiotic for urinary tract infection?

Trimethoprim or nitrofurantoin are recommended for first time presumed lower UTI in otherwise healthy women. In all other circumstances treatment should not be started until an MSU (plus blood culture if acute pyelonephritis is suspected) has been collected. Best guess antibiotics for lower UTI, acute pyelonephritis, urinary catheter sepsis and acute prostatitis are shown in Appendix 11. Note that these choices reflect the organisms prevalent in south west Scotland – they may be slightly different in other parts of the country. The choice of antibiotic should of course be reviewed once sensitivities are available.

Q12 What is an ESBL?

ESBL stands for Extended Spectrum Beta-Lactamase. ESBL is an enzyme produced by some E coli and some klebsiella. Its importance is that bacteria producing ESBL are resistant to many of the antibiotics commonly used for UTI. ESBL may be thought of as the gram negative equivalent of MRSA. In the case shown below the only antibiotics to which this particular organism was sensitive were meropenem and pivmecillinam (Fig. 31.2).

```
MG019499P            06/06/2012 21:00    Clean catch urine
Request Reason :     Known multiresistant Klebsiella UTI
                     Allergic to Penicillin and Erythromycin


Flow cytometry results –    see information below:-
WBC count                   3241        cells/uL
RBC count                   14          cells/uL
Epithelial cells count      32          cells/uL
Cast (Pathological) count   <0.2  cells/uL


WHITE CELL COUNT INTERPRETATION:    "0-39"   = not significant
                                    "40-89"  = +
                                    "90-599" = ++
                                    ">=600"  = +++


Culture:                                Auth
   1   Klebsiella pneumoniae (ESBL) >1x10^5 cfu/mL

   Amoxycillin          R      Meropenem          S
   Ciprofloxacin        R      Nitrofurantoin     R
   Co-amoxyclav         R      Pivmecillinam      S
   Gentamicin           R      Trimethoprim       R
```

Fig. 31.2 Example of ESBL organism cultured from urine sample

Q13 Should asymptomatic bacteriuria be treated with antibiotic?

The short answer is no. Asymptomatic bacteriuria increases with age and may affect up to 30 % of elderly men and women. Treatment with antibiotic does not improve urinary incontinence or reduce mortality. There is no evidence that asymptomatic bacteriuria causes renal scarring in adults. Exceptions to the 'don't treat' rule are pregnant women with asymptomatic bacteriuria who are otherwise at risk of ascending infection and acute pyelonephritis; recently transplanted kidney patients on high doses of immunosuppression; and possibly children with vesicoureteric reflux whose kidneys have not yet stopped growing.

Q14 Should catheter related urinary infection be treated with antibiotic?

Catheter associated infections should be treated but colonisation should not. Nearly all catheters become colonised by bacteria and treatment is best avoided in asymptomatic patients in order to reduce the risk of antibiotic resistance. You should not treat a change in colour or smell of the urine or a positive urinalysis result. Suspect catheter associated infection in a patient with one or more of fever ≥38.0 twice in 12 h, rigors, new delirium, loin or suprapubic tenderness and no other more likely source of infection. A CSU is then useful to determine the predominant organism and sensitivities. If a patient with a long term catheter develops a symptomatic UTI or gram negative septicaemia then it is important to change the catheter as well as treat with antibiotics.

Q15 What advice would you give to a woman with recurrent UTI?

Recurrent UTI are arbitrarily defined as three or more infections per year. The following simple advice may be helpful:
- Advise to drink 2 litres per day of fluid (not including tea or coffee).
- Empty bladder every 4 h.
- Remember to pass urine after intercourse.
- Consider cranberry. Cranberry juice has been shown to reduce risk of UTI but is not always to everyone's taste and one third of a litre is required each day. Powder and capsules can

provide higher concentrations and may be more palatable. Cranberry works by blocking adhesion of E.coli to epithelial cells within the urinary tract.

- Consider prophylactic antibiotic with single 200 mg dose of trimethoprim after intercourse if previous infections have been related to sex.

Q16   When would you recommend continuous antibiotic prophylaxis for patients with recurrent UTI?

Continuous prophylaxis should be considered for women who experience three or more symptomatic infections during a 12 month period or whenever the woman thinks that her life is being adversely affected by frequent recurrences. Antibiotics shown to be effective in this setting are given in Box 31.4.

Box 31.4 Prophylactic Doses of Antibiotic for Recurrent Urinary Tract Infection

Antibiotic	Dose	Frequency
Trimethoprim	100 mg	daily
Nitrofurantoin	50 or 100 mg	daily
Cefaclor	250 mg	daily
Cephalexin	125 or 250 mg	daily
Ciprofloxacin	125 mg	daily

It is customary to rotate these prophylactic antibiotics every 3 months and to stop after 6 months to see if the problem has resolved. If not then consider a longer course of rotating antibiotic for 1 year.

Q17   How often is 'confused and off legs' due to urosepsis?

Not as often as you might think. Elderly patients, usually elderly women, are frequently admitted to hospital with worsening confusion following a fall and incorrectly treated for urosepsis because their dipstick/urine culture was positive. The reality is that positive urine dipsticks and asymptomatic bacteriuria are so common in the elderly that they cannot be considered to be abnormal findings. If a patient can provide

a history then urosepsis can be confirmed if he or she has at least three acute symptoms e.g. dysuria, urgency, frequency or suprapubic symptoms together with a positive urine culture. If a patient cannot provide a history then urosepsis should only be diagnosed if there are features of systemic inflammation e.g. fever/hypothermia, raised WCC, raised CRP, plus a positive urine culture and no other more likely diagnosis.

Q18   What do you understand by the term pyonephrosis? How does it present and what should you do if suspected?

Literally pyonephrosis means pus in the kidney. Risk factors include structural disease such as an obstructing renal stone or pelviureteric junction obstruction or patients who are immunosuppressed by virtue of their diabetes or steroids. Pyonephrosis presents in the same way as acute pyelonephritis with loin pain, rigor and fever. The diagnosis should be suspected in patients who are particularly unwell from the outset or who don't respond to antibiotic, and is confirmed by ultrasound or CT. Pyonephrosis is a medical emergency that requires urgent drainage by nephrostomy or stenting in addition to broad spectrum antibiotic.

31.1   Objectives: Urinary Tract Infection

Q1   How does urinary tract infection present clinically?

Q2   Describe the typical clinical features of cystitis

Q3   What other causes of lower urinary tract symptoms do you know?

Q4   hat other diagnoses should you consider in patients with loin pain?

Q5   Which bacteria are most likely to cause UTI?

Q6   Give five important predisposing factors to UTI.

Q7   What is the role of the urine dipstick test in diagnosing urosepsis?

Q8   Is it always necessary to culture urine before starting antibiotics for suspected UTI?

Q9   What is the correct way to obtain a mid-stream specimen of urine (MSU)?

Q10 What if a patient who has been admitted to hospital with suspected UTI can't pass urine?

Q11 Which antibiotic for urinary tract infection?

Q12 What is an ESBL?

Q13 Should asymptomatic bacteriuria be treated with antibiotic?

Q14 Should catheter related urinary infection be treated with antibiotic?

Q15 What advice would you give to a woman with recurrent UTI?

Q16 When would you recommend continuous antibiotic prophylaxis for patients with recurrent UTI?

Q17 How often is 'confused and off legs' due to urosepsis?

Q18 What do you understand by the term pyonephrosis? How does it present and what should you do if suspected?

Further Reading

1. Management of suspected bacterial urinary tract infection in adults. SIGN Guideline 88. 2012. http://www.sign.ac.uk/guidelines/fulltext/88/index.html. Accessed 30 Sept 2014.
2. Ninan S, et al. Investigation of suspected urinary tract infection in older people. BMJ. 2014;348:g4070.

Q1 What are urinary stones and how commonly do they occur?

Urinary stones (calculi) are abnormal crystallized aggregates of common dietary minerals normally present in the urine. Calcium (as calcium oxalate or calcium phosphate) stones are by far the most common with urate, struvite and cystine calculi being less common. Lifetime risk is about 12 % in men and 6 % in women. The risk of recurrence with calcium stones is around 35–40 % at 5 years and 50 % at 10 years.

Box 32.1 Frequency of Urinary Stones

Composition	Frequency (%)
Calcium oxalate	60
Calcium phosphate	20
Magnesium ammonium phosphate (struvite)	5–10
Uric acid	5–10
Cystine	1

We devote the discussion that follows to stones that form in the kidney as opposed to stones that form in the ureter or bladder

Q2 How do urinary stones form?

The pathophysiology of renal stones varies, depending on the stone composition. Stones form when there is an excess of a particular substance, dehydration or an environment that is otherwise favourable to stone formation, as shown in Box 32.2.

Box 32.2 Pathophysiology and Stone Composition

Pathophysiology	Stone composition
"Supersaturation" of otherwise soluble material	Calcium, oxalate, phosphate, urate
Low urinary pH (acid urine)	Urate
Chronic/recurrent infections of upper urinary tract with urease producing bacteria	Struvite
Inherited defect of tubular resorption	Cystine

Q3 What medical diagnoses may be associated with stone formation?

Many systemic conditions can predispose patients to urinary stone disease. Prolonged hypercalcaemia of any cause (hyperparathyroidism, sarcoidosis, excessive dietary/prescribed calcium) results in larger than normal levels of excreted urinary calcium. Calcium oxalate stones may occur with any chronic diarrhea illness e.g. Crohn's disease. Calcium phosphate stones are associated with renal tubular acidosis, and urate stones with gout. Patients with recurrent/chronic urease producing bacterial infections of the upper urinary tract are at risk of struvite stones.

Q4 How do renal stones present?

Stone disease most commonly presents with renal, or more precisely ureteric, colic. Ureteric colic is an intense acute colicky loin pain with detectable haematuria, and often also with nausea,

M. Findlay, C. Isles, *Clinical Companion in Nephrology*,
DOI 10.1007/978-3-319-14868-7_32, © Springer International Publishing Switzerland 2015

vomiting, dysuria & urgency. The description of the pain can suggest the position of the stone with the common presentation of referred loin-to-groin pain suggesting the stone has travelled to the lower urinary tract and become lodged near the vesico-ureteric junction. Complications of an obstructing renal stone include infection and renal impairment though the latter can occur if stones are bilateral or the patient has only one kidney. Occasionally stones may be an incidental finding on a routine imaging procedure, or present as the painless passage of a small stone or gravel. Stones less than 6 mm diameter will usually pass spontaneously.

Q5   How would you investigate a patient with suspected ureteric colic?

The first presentation of renal stone disease is commonly as an "acute abdomen". Confirmation of the diagnosis is essential as other conditions may mimic renal colic – such as an ectopic pregnancy or leakage of an abdominal aortic aneurysm. A good history and a positive urinalysis for blood is suggestive but not diagnostic which means that imaging is required to confirm. Non contrast low radiation CT is now the investigation of choice for patients with acute flank pain. The combination of plain x-ray and ultrasound provides a cheaper alternative approach as 60 % urinary stones are radio-opaque and ultrasound can detect stones >5 mm diameter unless these have lodged in mid ureter. The advantage of CT is that it can exclude other important diagnoses while giving the clinician an idea of the size of the stone and therefore its likelihood of passage.

Q6   Describe the management of ureteric colic

NSAIDs and opiates are the mainstays of treatment. NSAIDs can be given orally or parenterally. Pethidine should be avoided because it commonly makes patients with ureteric colic vomit. Spontaneous passage rates can be increased by drugs that relax ureteric smooth muscle such as alpha blockers e.g. tamsulosin and calcium channel blockers e.g. nifedipine. Adequate hydration is important with most recommending 2 litres oral or IV intake per day. Relief of obstruction and treatment of infection may also be required.

Q7   What if the stone does not pass?

Emergency decompression by percutaneous nephrostomy or retrograde stent is indicated when stones obstruct a solitary kidney, with bilateral ureteric obstruction, for obstructed infected kidneys and for uncontrolled pain. Stones can then be fragmented by extracorporeal shock wave lithotripsy or retrieved by ureteroscopy. The advent of these minimally invasive interventions has dramatically reduced the need for open surgery.

Q8   What investigations should be undertaken to determine the cause of the stone?

The simplest approach is to request U&E including serum bicarbonate, serum calcium, phosphate and urate as a means of identifying patients with renal tubular acidosis, primary hyperparathyroidism and gout. A fresh urine sample may be sent for analysis for crystals (see below). Stones that pass spontaneously, are removed surgically, or excreted as fragments following disintegration, should be analysed to determine their composition. The added value of a 24 h urine collection for calcium, oxalate, urate and cystine is so low that we don't request this test routinely, though it does play a role in the further investigation of recurrent stone formers (Fig. 32.1).

Q9   What can be done to prevent calcium stones from recurring?

The following measures have been shown to reduce the risk of further calcium stones:
- Increased fluid intake to produce 2–3 litres of urine/day
- Reduced dietary intake of oxalate (e.g. rhubarb), animal protein and sodium
- Treatment with thiazides

It is generally agreed that prevention should start with advice regarding dietary and drinking habits, reserving thiazides for patients in whom the non-pharmacological measures fail. Note that dietary calcium intake should not be restricted because calcium binds oxalate in the gut and low calcium diet may therefore lead to increased oxalate absorption. We summarise advice for calcium and other stones in the box below. For more detailed recommendations see the European Association of Urology guidelines (referenced below)

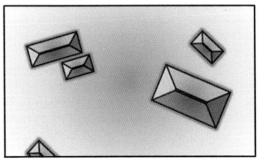

Struvite

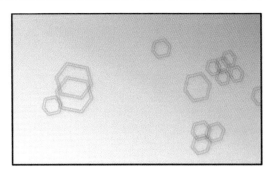

Cystine

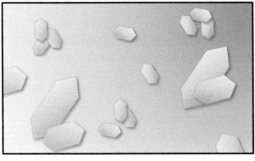

Urate

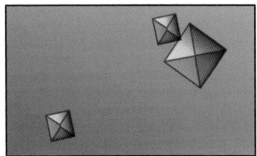

Oxalate

Fig. 32.1 Microscopic appearance of urinary crystals

Box 32.3 Targeted Medical Therapies for Stone Disease

Drink plenty to maintain high urine output

Maintain good calcium intake but do not take calcium supplements

Consider thiazide for hypercalciuria

Allopurinol to dissolve urate stones

Penicillamine to dissolve cystine stones

Alkalinise urine for urate & cystine stones

32.1 Objectives: Renal Stone Disease

Q1 What are urinary stones and how commonly do they occur?

Q2 How do urinary stones form?

Q3 What medical diagnoses may be associated with stone formation?

Q4 How do renal stones present?

Q5 How would you investigate a patient with suspected ureteric colic?

Q6 Describe the management of ureteric colic

Q7 What if the stone does not pass?

Q8 What investigations should be undertaken to determine the cause of the stone?

Q9 What can be done to prevent calcium stones from recurring?

Further Reading

1. Bultitude M, Rees J. Management of renal colic. BMJ. 2012;345:e5499.
2. Tiselius H-G, et al. Guidelines on Urolithiasis. European Association of Urology. 2009. http://www.uroweb.org/fileadmin/tx_eauguidelines/2008/Full/17%20Urolithiasis.p.

Q1 How common is chronic pain in renal disease?

Pain is a common problem affecting 10–25 % of the general population. Studies suggest that at least 50 % patients with severe CKD (eGFR <30 ml/min) including patients on dialysis experience chronic pain. The high prevalence of pain is concerning because pain adversely affects quality of life.

Q2 What are the likely causes of pain in a patient with CKD?

There are a wide variety of causes of pain in CKD and dialysis patients. Some are specific to kidney patients but most are not. Whatever the cause of pain this is likely to increase in intensity during dialysis. This is at least partly because patients cannot move around to ease their pain, and partly because opioid drugs are cleared from the circulation during dialysis. Pain in dialysis patients can be classified as follows:

Box 33.1 Causes of Pain in Dialysis Patients
Pain specific to renal patients

Hand pain due to vascular steal in a fistula arm.

Cyst pain in polycystic kidneys.

Pain of calciphylaxis – calciphylaxis is the term used to describe the skin necrosis that occurs in some patients with uncontrolled secondary hyperparathyroidism.

Neuropathic pain

Critical limb ischaemia

Phantom limb pain after amputation.

Limb pain from peripheral neuropathy e.g. diabetic neuropathy.

Sciatica.

Non neuropathic pain

Degenerative back pain.

Pain of intermittent claudication.

Pain from osteoporotic vertebral fractures.

Bone pain from myelomatous deposits

Q3 Describe in broad terms your approach to chronic pain in a patient with CKD.

First, you should investigate this unless it has already been investigated. For example if a CKD patient complains of back pain, degenerative changes and osteoporotic fractures are more common than myelomatous deposits but all three need to be considered. Next you must appreciate that the answer to pain does not always lie in a bottle of tablets. People's perception of pain, and learned responses to pain vary enormously. The psyche contributes significantly to the severity of pain and its impact on a patient's life. At one extreme exists the patient who stubs a toe and attends for a sick line, while at the other extreme there are patients who live with chronic inflammatory or malignant pain, and still continue to hold down jobs. Having said all that, it is likely that most patients with chronic pain will require some form of analgesia.

> Managing chronic pain requires exploration and management of both the underlying physical and psychological components of an individual's pain syndrome.

Q4 Does the Analgesic Ladder work in CKD patients?

Yes. In 1986 the WHO established an evidence based three step ladder for mild (1–3/10 pain score), moderate (4–6/10) and severe (>7/10) levels of malignant pain that has since been adapted for other patient groups including CKD and ESRD patients (Fig. 33.1).

At any step in the ladder adjuvant drugs may be added depending on the cause of the pain. These include antidepressants and anticonvulsant drugs for neuropathic pain.

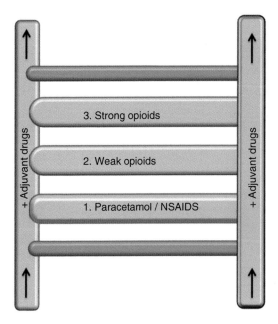

Fig. 33.1 The WHO analgesic ladder

Q5 What place is there for paracetamol for chronic pain in CKD?

Paracetamol does not accumulate in renal failure but may be nephrotoxic if given at very high doses/in overdose. The dose of paracetamol for predialysis patients is the same as for normal renal function while dialysis patients are safe to receive paracetamol as first line treatment for pain up to a maximum of 1G three times daily

Q6 What place is there for non steroidal anti-inflammatory drugs for chronic pain in CKD?

Non steroidal anti-inflammatory drugs increase the risk of GI bleeding in dialysis patients and are also nephrotoxic, as shown in Box 33.2. NSAIDs should probably be avoided in patients with eGFR less than 60 ml/min because of this. They can however be used with caution for short periods if the doctor and patient are prepared to monitor their effects on the kidney closely. It could be argued that once a patient is on dialysis then NSAIDs can be used again on the grounds that they have no more renal function to lose. This is certainly true of the anuric patient, but may not be true for patients with significant residual renal function. Finally, there are no advantages to giving COX-2 inhibitors (such as celecoxib) to renal patients. They are just as nephrotoxic as NSAIDs

> **Box 33.2 Nephrotoxic Effects of NSAIDs**
> • Reversible acute renal failure because they inhibit the enzyme that produces the prostaglandins which dilate the afferent arteriole.
> • Sodium and water retention.
> • Hyperkalaemia.
> • Aggravate hypertension.
> • Interstitial nephritis.
> • Minimal change nephrotic syndrome.

Q7 Discuss the role of codeine and tramadol for chronic pain in patients with CKD.

The step 2 drugs are weak opioids for mild to moderate pain e.g. codeine and tramadol±non opioid analgesics±adjuvant drugs. Codeine and tramadol are both metabolised by the liver, but have active metabolites that are excreted by the kidney. They are not nephrotoxic but both are more likely to cause opiate toxicity in a renal patient than in a patient with normal renal function. The dose of both drugs should be reduced when GFR falls below 30 ml/min. Most recommend that codeine be avoided in dialysis patients and that low doses of tramadol be used with caution (see Appendix 15)

Cocodamol, which contains both paracetamol and codeine, is often prescribed for patients with chronic pain. It comes in two strengths: 30/500 containing 30 mg of codeine and 8/500 containing 8 mg of codeine. Both preparations contain 500 mg paracetamol. Cocodamol 8/500 is therefore preferred when eGFR is less than 30 ml/min. In addition, it is best to prescribe Cocodamol tablets that are swallowed whole rather than effervescent tablets. Eight tablets of Cocodamol effervescent per day contains 148 mmol sodium which is enough additional sodium to cause a dialysis patient to become hypertensive or retain fluid.

Q8 Which step 3 drugs are preferred for patients with advanced CKD and chronic pain and why?

Step 3 drugs are strong opioids for severe pain±non opioid analgesics±adjuvants. Oral morphine should be used with caution when GFR falls below 30 ml/min because of its active metabolite morphine-6-glucuronide which is renally excreted and causes opioid toxicity especially drowsiness, myoclonic twitching and hallucinations. Oral oxycodone is better tolerated than morphine but also best avoided except when given as oxynorm for breakthrough. Fentanyl and alfentanil are preferred to morphine and oxycodone in haemodialysis patients for the following reasons. Transdermal fentanyl is metabolised mainly in the liver which means that the dose used in patients with renal failure can be exactly the same as the dose used for someone with normal renal function. Fentanyl toxicity from too high a dose is subtler than morphine toxicity due to lack of hallucinations and myoclonus, and may present instead as vagueness, drowsiness or 'not feeling well'. Subcutaneous alfentanil is metabolised by the liver, like fentanyl. Its onset of action is more rapid than for fentanyl. Alfentanil's analgesic effect lasts for around 2 h which means it can either be used for breakthrough pain or in a syringe driver. For doses in severe CKD and dialysis patients, see Appendix 15

Q9 Describe the symptoms of opiate toxicity.

Constipation is universal while nausea and vomiting occur in at least 50 %. The side effects of opiates may usefully be considered as follows:

Box 33.3 Symptoms of Opioid Toxicity	
There are three groups of symptoms, namely:	
1. Gastrointestinal	Constipation is universal while nausea and vomiting occur in at least 50 %.
2. Autonomic nervous system	Dry mouth, sweating.
3. Central nervous system	Drowsiness, confusion, hallucination, myoclonus (muscle jerks) and respiratory depression.

Q10 What steps might you take to reduce the risk of constipation and nausea when starting a patient with severe CKD on an opiate for chronic pain?

First, use a fentanyl patch rather than morphine or oxycodone. Second, a pre-emptive approach is best. Laxatives should be prescribed whenever an opiate is started. Anti-emetics are needed in 50–75 % of patients on strong opioids. Metoclopramide, haloperidol, cyclizine and ondansetron are all effective in opiate toxicity. Metoclopramide should be used with caution as there is a greater risk of facial dyskinesia. Haloperidol reduces seizure threshold and should be avoided in patients with a history of epilepsy. Cyclizine may induce hypotension and tachyarrythmia and is not generally recommended in dialysis patients. Regular ondansetron can relieve itch but may cause constipation. The dose of metoclopramide and haloperidol should be reduced in renal failure, whereas no dose reduction is necessary for the other two drugs. Dosing schedules for severe CKD and dialysis patients are given in Appendix 15.

Q11 How would you manage a diabetic dialysis patient with chronic back pain who has just been started on oxycodone and who is drowsy with shallow respirations when brought in for dialysis?

Decreased conscious level with respiratory upset must be managed as with all medical emergencies – using the ABCDE approach. Ensure that you check blood glucose to rule out hypoglycaemia prior to treating for opioid toxicity. If blood glucose is normal, give naloxone, in increments of 100 micrograms to a total of 400 micrograms IV. If no response this can be repeated until a total of 2 mg has been given. Naloxone reverses all the effects of opiates (including pain control) and most opiate toxic patients will respond pretty quickly when naloxone is given. If there is no response to a total of 2 mg IV then it is unlikely that opiates are responsible for their drowsiness or shallow breaths. If naloxone works then you may need to start a naloxone infusion and continue this for up to 48 h if a dialysis patient has been taking oxycodone, as

the half life of this drug in advanced renal failure is very much prolonged.

Q12 How would you manage a dialysis patient with chronic back pain on a 50 mcg/h Fentanyl patch whose pain is normally well controlled but who experiences much more severe back pain while on dialysis?

Patients with chronic pain may need 'breakthrough' analgesia or 'rescue doses' during dialysis. This should be in the form of a strong opioid. In this scenario, the logical drug to give is alfentanil SC or IV, the dose of which should be determined by consulting your Palliative Care Unit's pain chart. You could also use oramorph orally for this purpose though you would need to bear in mind that the effects of oramorph will last a little longer than usual because its active metabolite is renally excreted.

Q13 What might make you think that a patient was experiencing neuropathic pain?

Neuropathic (nerve) pain is characteristically burning, shooting or stabbing. It often occurs in an area of abnormal sensation and may be associated with hyperalgesia and allodynia (pain from a stimulus that is not normally painful). Examples of neuropathic pain include the pain of peripheral neuropathy and the pain of limb ischaemia.

Q14 Describe the drug therapy of neuropathic pain in dialysis patients.

The drugs available for neuropathic pain include the tricyclic antidepressant, amitriptyline and the anti-convulsant drugs carbamazepine, valproate and gabapentin. The only one of these to require a dose reduction in renal failure is gabapentin. Suggested dosing schedules for a dialysis patient are given in Appendix 15

33.1 Objectives: Managing Pain in Chronic Kidney Disease

After reading this chapter, you should be able to answer the following:

Q1 How common is chronic pain in dialysis patients?

Q2 What are the likely causes of pain in a patient with CKD?

Q3 Describe in broad terms your approach to chronic pain in patients with CKD

Q4 Does the Analgesic Ladder work in CKD patients?

Q5 What place is there for paracetamol for chronic pain in CKD patients?

Q6 What place is there for non steroidal anti-inflammatory drugs for chronic pain in CKD?

Q7 Discuss the role of codeine and tramadol for chronic pain in patients CKD.

Q8 Which step 3 drugs are preferred for patients with advances CKD and chronic pain and why?

Q9 Describe the symptoms of opiate toxicity.

Q10 What steps might you take to reduce the risk of constipation and nausea when starting a patient with severe CKD on an opiate for chronic pain?

Q11 How would you manage a diabetic dialysis patient with chronic back pain who has just been started on oxycodone and who is drowsy with shallow respirations when brought in for dialysis?

Q12 How would you manage a dialysis patient with chronic back pain on a 50 mcg/h Fentanyl patch whose pain is normally well controlled but who experiences much more severe back pain while on dialysis?

Q13 What might make you think that a patient was experiencing neuropathic pain?

Q14 Describe the drug therapy of neuropathic pain in dialysis patients.

Further Reading

1. Pham P-C, et al. Pain management in chronic kidney disease. NDT Plus. 2009;2:111–8.
2. Scottish Palliative Care Guidelines, Health improvement Scotland. 2014. www.palliativecareguidelines.scot.nhs.uk.

Q1 Describe the changes in renal physiology that occur in normal pregnancy.

'In pregnancy everything gets bigger'. Both kidneys increase in size by 1–2 cm. GFR increases by up to 50 % in the second trimester. There is a corresponding fall in serum creatinine which therefore becomes a less useful marker of acute kidney injury i.e. a pregnant patient can lose 50 % of her renal function and still have serum creatinine that is well within the normal range. Hormonal and pressure effects cause dilatation of the ureters and renal pelvis which is often more marked on the right side, from the second trimester onwards. This increases the risk of ascending infection (Fig. 34.1).

Q2 What effect does pregnancy have on the kidney?

The risk of ascending urinary infection is increased for the reasons given above. Acute pyelonephritis occurs in up to 25 % pregnant women with asymptomatic bacteriuria and because of this antibiotic treatment is indicated. More importantly there is a risk that renal function will deteriorate that is related to serum creatinine concentration at the start of pregnancy. Renal function hardly ever deteriorates if baseline creatinine is less than 125 μmol/l but frequently does if baseline creatinine is higher than this (Box 34.1). Patients with proteinuric nephropathy will almost always develop heavier proteinuria during pregnancy. For some this may

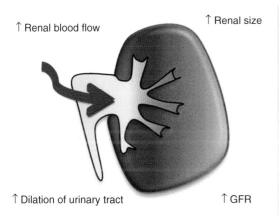

↑ Renal blood flow   ↑ Renal size

↑ Dilation of urinary tract   ↑ GFR

Fig. 34.1 Changes to kidney structure and function during pregnancy

Box 34.1 Predicted Renal Outcomes Following Pregnancy in Those with Underlying CKD

Pre-pregnancy creatinine (μmol/L)	Loss of >25 % renal function during pregnancy (%)	Progression to ESRF after 1 year (%)
<125	2	0
125–180	40	2
>180	70	35

Reproduced from Chronic kidney disease in pregnancy, Williams D and Davidson J, *BMJ* 2008; 336:211–5 with permission from BMJ Publishing Group Ltd

M. Findlay, C. Isles, *Clinical Companion in Nephrology*,
DOI 10.1007/978-3-319-14868-7_34, © Springer International Publishing Switzerland 2015

mean nephrotic range proteinuria leading to significant oedema. Proteinuria tends to return to baseline values after delivery.

Q3   What effect does chronic kidney disease have on pregnancy outcome?

Fertility falls as creatinine rises which means that conception becomes progressively less likely as GFR declines. When pregnancy does occur the presence of CKD results in increased risk of gestational hypertension, pre-eclampsia, eclampsia, intra-uterine growth retardation, premature birth and both foetal and maternal death. The diagnosis of pre-eclampsia is made more difficult if both proteinuria and hypertension are present in the first trimester.

Q4   What advice would you give to a young female attending the general renal clinic who wishes to become pregnant?

It is important to inform her of the risks of the pregnancy to her renal function and the risks of her renal function to the pregnancy. Review her medication – changing antihypertensive therapy to safer alternatives where possible. ACE inhibitors/ARBs should be discontinued, although exceptional circumstances exist in which those with very high proteinuria, the possibility of a prolonged time period before pregnancy and a reliable method of early pregnancy detection, may remain on these drugs until pregnancy is confirmed. It is worth remembering, however, that the risk from ACE inhibitors/ARBs is highest during the period of organogenesis (i.e., the first trimester). Folic acid 5 mg od should be prescribed as should aspirin 75 mg od, which may reduce the risk of pre-eclampsia.

Q5   How often do dialysis patients become pregnant?

Not very often. Most women on dialysis are beyond childbearing age and younger dialysis patients are likely to be less sexually active than their non renal counterparts. Menstruation on dialysis is likely to be absent, irregular or anovulatory. Spontaneous miscarriage is perhaps the commonest outcome for a dialysis patient who becomes pregnant while prematurity and intra-uterine

growth retardation are ever present risks for those pregnancies that do not abort.

Q6   What should you tell a patient on dialysis who wishes to become pregnant?

Where possible to wait until she has a well-functioning renal transplant. If she does become pregnant while on dialysis the literature suggests that a live birth will only occur in 30–50 % of pregnancies. From a practical point of view pregnant haemodialysis patients should dialyse with a left lateral head up tilt to optimise blood flow and so prevent sudden drops in blood pressure. The best hope for a healthy baby is to follow the advice given in the box below.

Box 34.2 Advice to Optimise Pregnancy Outcomes in Patients on Haemodialysis
1. Intensive dialysis, aiming to maintain pre-dialysis urea <17 mmol/l.
2. Prevention of maternal hypotension.
3. Improvement in maternal nutrition.
4. Management of anaemia.
5. Correction of acidosis and hypocalcaemia.
6. Foetal monitoring from week 24 onwards.

Q7   What effect does renal transplantation have on fertility?

Transplant patients of child bearing age should be advised that fertility can return rapidly. It is normally recommended that patients do not become pregnant for 1 year (living related) or 2 years (cadaveric) following transplantation. This is to give sufficient time to stabilise the patient on immunosuppressive drugs and so minimise the risk of future graft dysfunction. For planned pregnancies, modify the immunosuppression so as to avoid sirolimus (rapamycin) and mycophenolate mofetil (MMF) both of which may cause foetal malformation. The combination of tacrolimus and prednisolone with or without azathioprine is usually recommended.

Q8   AKI in pregnancy is uncommon. Discuss.

AKI was relatively common in the 1960s but nowadays rarely complicates pregnancy. In early pregnancy the risk factors are similar to those for non-pregnant women, for example volumes losses due to hyperemesis or sepsis related to septic abortion. An important and difficult differential diagnosis is that of AKI in the third trimester in association with microangiopathic hemolytic anemia and thrombocytopenia. The two important differential diagnoses to consider are HUS-TTP and the Haemolysis Elevated Liver Enzymes Low Platelets (HELLP) variant of severe pre-eclampsia. It is important to differentiate one from the other and seek expert help early as the management strategies are very different. For more detailed discussion of this topic we suggest the article on AKI in Pregnancy in UpToDate (referenced at the end of this chapter).

34.1   Objectives: Pregnancy and Renal Disease

After reading this chapter, you should be able to answer the following:

Q1   Describe the changes in renal physiology that occur in normal pregnancy

Q2   What effect does pregnancy have on the kidney?

Q3   What effect does chronic kidney disease have on pregnancy outcome?

Q4   What advice would you give to a young female attending the general renal clinic who wishes to become pregnant?

Q5   How often do dialysis patients become pregnant?

Q6   What should you tell a patient on dialysis who wishes to become pregnant?

Q7   What effect does renal transplantation have on fertility?

Q8   AKI in pregnancy is uncommon. Discuss.

Further Reading

1. UpToDate: Acute Kidney Injury in Pregnancy. www.uptodate.com/contents/acute-kidney-injury-acute-renal-failure-in-pregnancy. Accessed 25 Sept 2014.
2. Williams D, Davison J. Chronic kidney disease in pregnancy. BMJ. 2008;336:211–5.

Q1 Which blood borne virus (BBV) infections are recognised as hazards for patients and staff in Renal Units?

There are three: hepatitis B virus (HBV), hepatitis C virus (HCV) and human immunodeficiency virus (HIV). The main risks relate to HBV outbreaks due to the greater chance of infection from needle-stick injury, its chronic carrier state and the virus' ability to survive for up to 7 days on environmental surfaces. HCV and HIV are less infectious in dialysis units, though outbreaks have been reported emphasising the need for infection control measures.

Q2 Give the routes of transmission, clinical presentation and treatment options for HBV.

HBV is the most likely of the BBV to be transmitted by needle-stick injury, with a risk that may be as high as 1 in 3 if the infected patient is eAntigen positive or has a high viral load. HBV can also be transmitted sexually, from mother to child ("vertical transmission") and rarely via blood transfusions. Figure 35.1 shows worldwide prevalence. The ability of this virus to survive outside the human body causes concern in renal units because of "horizontal transmission" – patient to patient. Presentation is usually with jaundice and raised transaminases. Diagnosis is confirmed if patient is HBsAg positive and becomes antiHBs/anti-HBc positive. Viral load and is quantified by HBV-DNA. HBV can be prevented by vaccination and treated but not cured with suppressive therapy.

Q3 Give the routes of transmission, clinical presentation and treatment options for HCV.

The majority of HCV infection is related to IV drug abuse or blood transfusion. However, blood transfusion accounts for far fewer cases than in the past since the introduction of viral screening in 1991. Sexual transmission is low. The risk of acquiring HCV from a needlestick injury is around 1 in 30. Infected patients are less likely to present with jaundice than HBV and are more commonly detected by screening or during investigation of abnormal LFTs. The diagnosis is confirmed if the patient is HCV-PCR positive and anti-HCV positive. Viral load is then quantified by the HCV-QPCR test. There is no vaccine for HCV but cure rates of up to 95 % can now be expected with the latest treatments.

Q4 Give the routes of transmission, clinical presentation and treatment options for HIV.

HIV is usually transmitted sexually. It has been reported in all risk categories particularly men who have sex with men (MSM), but also intravenous drug abusers, recipients of blood transfusion and needlestick injuries. Heterosexual transmission may occur. The risk of HIV from a needlestick injury is around 1 in 300. Over 50 % of patients will be symptomatic in early infection but symptoms are often non-specific – sore throat, lymphadenopathy, fever and rash – and may not be reported. Therefore patients are either

M. Findlay, C. Isles, *Clinical Companion in Nephrology*,
DOI 10.1007/978-3-319-14868-7_35, © Springer International Publishing Switzerland 2015

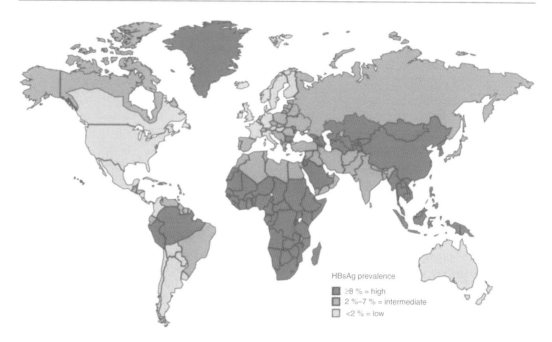

Fig. 35.1 Worldwide prevalence of hepatitis B surface antigen, 2006 (Reproduced with permission from US Centres of Disease Control, http://www.cdc.gov/hepatitis/HBV/PDFs/HBV_figure3map_08-27-08.pdf)

picked up by screening or when they develop AIDS. A diagnosis of HIV infection is made in patients who are HIV antigen/antibody positive. Their viral load is then quantified by HIV-RNA testing. There is no vaccine and no cure but highly active anti-retroviral treatment (HAART) is both disease suppressive and life prolonging.

Q5   What measures should routinely be taken by staff to prevent BBV transmission?

Measures to prevent BBV transmission are those that effectively prevent the transfer of blood or fluids contaminated with blood between patients or staff either directly or via contaminated equipment or surfaces. Hand-washing, avoidance of cross-contamination, appropriate cleaning protocols and safe disposal of waste are key.

Q6   To what extent can transmission of BBV be prevented by vaccination?

At present we only have a vaccine for HBV. Vaccine is given at 0, 1 and 6 months (HBvaxPRO 40ug) or at 0, 1, 2 and 6 months (Engerix B 40ug) and the antibody titre is checked to assess for a response. Antibody responses to hepatitis B vaccine vary widely between individuals and while it is best to achieve anti-HBs levels above 100 IU/L it is generally accepted that levels over 10 IU/L will offer

some protection against infection. Patients with antibody levels 10–99 IU/L are offered a fourth dose of vaccine. All patients who are likely to require renal replacement therapy should be identified, whenever possible, early in the course of their disease and vaccinated. All staff who have clinical contact with patients should be immunised against HBV and demonstrate immunity (Fig. 35.2).

Q7   How often should dialysis patients be screened for BBV?

The Renal Association recommend regular, routine testing for hepatitis B surface antigen (HBsAg), HCV antibody & HIV antibody in all patients being treated in a haemodialysis unit.

> **Box 35.1 Renal Association Guidelines for Screening of BBV**
>
> **Hepatitis B** – Varies with response to vaccination. Test for HBsAg in responders yearly and non-responders at least every 3 months.
>
> **HCV** – test for HCV antibody at least every 6 months.
>
> **HIV** – Routine testing not recommended unless "high risk". (See further reading)

Fig. 35.2 Flowchart for
hepatitis B vaccination

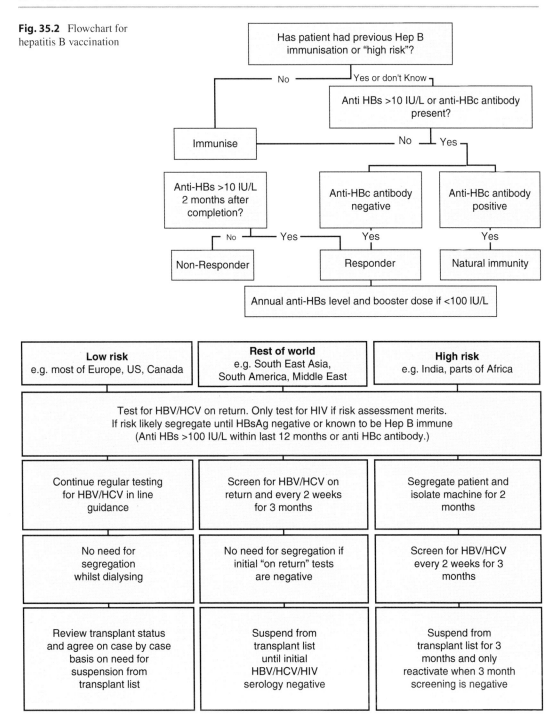

Low risk e.g. most of Europe, US, Canada	Rest of world e.g. South East Asia, South America, Middle East	High risk e.g. India, parts of Africa
Test for HBV/HCV on return. Only test for HIV if risk assessment merits. If risk likely segregate until HBsAg negative or known to be Hep B immune (Anti HBs >100 IU/L within last 12 months or anti HBc antibody.)		
Continue regular testing for HBV/HCV in line guidance	Screen for HBV/HCV on return and every 2 weeks for 3 months	Segregate patient and isolate machine for 2 months
No need for segregation whilst dialysing	No need for segregation if initial "on return" tests are negative	Screen for HBV/HCV every 2 weeks for 3 months
Review transplant status and agree on case by case basis on need for suspension from transplant list	Suspend from transplant list until initial HBV/HCV/HIV serology negative	Suspend from transplant list for 3 months and only reactivate when 3 month screening is negative

Fig. 35.3   Algorithm of BBV management for patients recently dialysing elsewhere

Q8   What additional precautions are necessary in patients returning after holiday dialysis and in visitors from other units?

All patients and machines should be segregated until known to be HBsAg, HCV antibody and HCV-PCR negative by applying the following algorithm (Fig. 35.3).

35.1   Objectives: Blood Borne Viruses

After reading this chapter you should be able to answer the following:

Q1 Which blood borne virus (BBV) infections are recognised as hazards for patients and staff in Renal Units?

Q2 Give the routes of transmission, clinical presentation and treatment options for HBV.

Q3 Give the routes of transmission, clinical presentation and treatment options for HCV.

Q4 Give the routes of transmission, clinical presentation and treatment options for HIV.

Q5 What measures should routinely be taken by staff to prevent BBV transmission?

Q6 To what extent can transmission of BBV be prevented by vaccination?

Q7 How often should dialysis patients be screened for BBV?

Q8 What additional precautions are necessary in patients returning after holiday dialysis and in visitors from other units?

Further Reading

1. Geddes C, Lindley E, Duncan N. Renal Association Clinical Practice Guidelines – Blood Borne Virus Infection. 2009. Access via www.renal.org.

Q1 What is reflux nephropathy and how is it treated?

Previously called chronic pyelonephritis, reflux nephropathy is a form of interstitial renal disease that may be the cause of around 10 % of the CKD in UK patients who require dialysis. The aetiology is thought to be vesico-ureteric reflux (VUR) combined with ascending infection in early life, leading to renal inflammation with cortical scars and calyceal clubbing. Historically the diagnosis was made by IVP, showing a triad of small irregular kidneys with cortical scars and calyceal clubbing. Nowadays, ultrasound will pick up major anatomical abnormalities but early scars are best detected by DMSA isotope scan. Those with hypertension, proteinuria and bilateral disease are more likely to progress to ESRD than those without these risk factors and whose serum creatinine is normal. In adulthood treatment is conservative with prompt management of underlying symptomatic infection.

Q2 How does lupus affect the kidney and how is this treated?

Renal disease is common in SLE with up to 75 % of all those with SLE developing some evidence of renal involvement during their lifetime. Six distinct pathological entities are described ranging from minimal evidence of immune deposition to more active focal or diffuse disease (+/– crescentic lesions) or advanced sclerosis. The clinical presentation of lupus nephritis invariably involves proteinuria, which may be in the nephrotic range. Other presentations include haematuria, hypertension and deteriorating renal function including RPGN. Signs of renal involvement with evidence of a high anti-DNA and low complement titre (C3/C4) are suggestive of active lupus nephritis, although a renal biopsy is required to achieve a diagnosis and plan management. Management of active disease is largely based on immunosuppression with steroids, mycophenolate +/– cyclophosphamide.

Q3 What is renal amyloidosis and how is it treated?

Amyloidosis is a complex group of acquired or inherited conditions characterised by extracellular deposition of an abnormal protein (amyloid fibrils) within various body tissues. Acquired amyloidosis, specifically AA (secondary) and AL (primary) amyloidosis, commonly presents with renal disease. Proteinuria is common, renal impairment less so and tubular dysfunction rare. AA amyloidosis is associated with chronic inflammatory disorders such as bronchiectasis, osteitis and chronic tuberculosis. Treatment is directed at the underlying inflammation, supplemented by best supportive CKD care. Renal prognosis is poor with patients often developing ESRF. However, in those who receive a transplant, graft survival is similar to the general population. AL amyloidosis is a plasma cell disorder, similar to myeloma, which results in an excess of abnormal immunoglobulin light chains. Chemotherapy is used to lower the light chain burden.

M. Findlay, C. Isles, *Clinical Companion in Nephrology*,
DOI 10.1007/978-3-319-14868-7_36, © Springer International Publishing Switzerland 2015

Q4   What is medullary sponge kidney and how is it treated?

Medullary sponge kidney is usually a benign condition, characterised by malformed, dilated collecting ducts which result in the formation of medullary cysts of various sizes. It is thought to be a developmental abnormality, and may cluster in families. For most this condition remains asymptomatic with preserved excretory renal function. However recurrent haematuria, urinary tract infections or renal stone disease may be a presenting feature in some and, if complicated, can lead to deterioration in renal function. Plain x-ray and ultrasound often suggests nephrocalcinosis but both may be falsely negative. Intravenous pyelogram (IVP) was always the investigation of choice, showing a radial, linear or "brush like" pattern in the papillae with contrast medium in the ectatic collecting ducts seen as a "bouquet of flowers". Nowadays CT urography may be preferred. Therapy is aimed at managing complications such as urinary tract infection or stone disease.

Q5   How does HIV affect the kidney and how is it treated?

With the overall improvement in life expectancy, conditions such as chronic kidney disease, hypertension and diabetes add to the long term disease burden. There are two unique causes of renal disease in patients with HIV: directly as a result of HIV infection or indirectly from use of anti-retroviral therapies. The latter presents as stone disease or electrolyte disturbance (including Fanconi's syndrome) and is managed as for the general population. HIV associated nephropathy (HIVAN) usually presents with nephrotic range proteinuria and may progress to renal failure. The most common renal lesion on biopsy is a focal glomerulosclerosis. Treatment is that of the underlying disease with HAART which can stabilise and even reverse the renal failure.

Q6   What is the Fanconi syndrome and how is it treated?

This rare renal disease is a disorder of proximal tubular function, characterised by the combination of low serum phosphate, potassium and bicarbonate with glycosuria and amino aciduria. This collection of defects indicates diffuse involvement of the proximal tubule rather than a single channel defect. Causes may be inherited (usually as part of another condition) or acquired (toxins, myeloma or transplantation). Inherited Fanconi's presents in childhood with polyuria, polydipsia, impaired growth and rickets. Presentation is similar in adults but it may also come to light during investigation of hypokalaemia and acidosis. Treatment is targeted at the underlying cause and replacement of deficiencies.

Q7   What inherited syndromes may cause hypokalaemia with metabolic alkalosis?

There are three: Bartter's, Gitelman's and Liddle's syndromes. All three are rare with most clinicians only coming across them when studying for professional exams. These inherited conditions are caused by specific channel defects within the tubule. Barrter's and Gitelman's syndromes are salt losing with low or normal blood pressure whereas Liddle's syndrome is salt retaining with high blood pressure. A summary of differences between each condition is given in Table 36.1. For advice on treatment see www.rarerenal.org

Q8   How does sarcoidosis affect the kidney and how is this treated?

Sarcoidosis is a multisystem inflammatory granulomatous condition of unknown aetiology characterised by presence of non-caseating granulomata in various organs. Renal disease can occasionally complicate sarcoidosis although the incidence of renal involvement is unknown. Hypercalcaemia – a common finding in sarcoidosis – predisposes to polyuria, nephrolithiasis and nephrocalcinosis. Renal stone disease may be the presenting feature of sarcoidosis. Sarcoidosis-related interstitial nephritis is more likely to present at the time of diagnosis and rarely complicates long standing sarcoidosis. Treatment predominantly consists of steroids. End-stage renal failure requiring long term dialysis is uncommon.

Table 36.1 Tubular channelopathies

	Barrter's syndrome	Gitelman's syndrome	Liddle's syndrome
Age at presentation	Childhood	Adulthood	Childhood
Blood pressure	Low/normal	Low/normal	High
Inheritance	Autosomal recessive	Autosomal recessive	Autosomal dominant
Channel	Na-K-2Cl (TAL)	Na-Cl (DCT)	ENaC (CD)
Serum K	Low	Low	Low
Serum Bicarbonate	High	High	High
Serum Magnesium	Normal	Low	Normal
Urine calcium	High	Low	Normal
Diuretic mimic	Loop	Thiazide	

36.1   Objectives: Rarer Renal Diseases

After reading this chapter, you should be able to answer the following:

Q1   What is reflux nephropathy and how is it treated?

Q2   How does lupus affect the kidney and how is this treated?

Q3   What is renal amyloidosis and how is it treated?

Q4   What is medullary sponge kidney and how is it treated?

Q5   How does HIV affect the kidney and how is it treated?

Q6   What is the Fanconi syndrome and how is it treated?

Q7   What inherited syndromes may cause hypokalaemia with metabolic alkalosis?

Q8   How does sarcoidosis affect the kidney and how is this treated?

Further Reading

1. For details of other rarer renal diseases such as Alport's syndrome, cystinosis, cystinuria, hyperoxaluria, pure red cell aplasia go to the Renal Association website. http://www.rarerenal.org.

Part VI

Renal Replacement Therapy

Haemodialysis

Q1 Describe the different types of renal replacement therapy.

There are three. These are haemodialysis, peritoneal dialysis and transplantation. Haemodialysis may be undertaken in hospital or at home. Peritoneal dialysis is always done at home either during the day (Continuous Ambulatory Peritoneal Dialysis or CAPD) or overnight (Automated Peritoneal Dialysis or APD). Transplantation may either be by cadaveric or live donor. Conservative care is a further treatment option for patients with end stage renal disease and may well be the appropriate form of treatment for the frail elderly with multiple co-morbidities. PD, transplantation and conservative care are discussed in more detail in the chapters that follow.

Q2 How many patients receiving RRT will be on haemodialysis, peritoneal dialysis or have a functioning transplant?

The take on rate for renal replacement therapy appears to be plateauing at around 100 patients per million per year in the UK, though higher take on rates are seen in those parts of the country with significant Black African and Asian communities. Good pre-dialysis education is nowadays usually possible for all except those who present acutely, and means that patients are able to weigh up the pros and cons of each type of treatment and then make an informed decision. Latest UK figures from December 2012 suggest that despite efforts to promote PD, 86 % of dialysis patients (43 % of the total RRT population) will end up

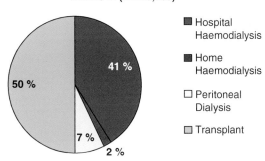

Prevalent RRT patients in UK Dec 2012 (n = 55,000)

- ■ Hospital Haemodialysis
- ■ Home Haemodialysis
- ☐ Peritoneal Dialysis
- ☐ Transplant

41 %

50 %

7 %

2 %

Fig. 37.1 UK prevalence by RRT modality UK Renal Registry, The Sixteenth Annual Report, 2013

doing HD and only 14 % of dialysis patients (7 % of the total RRT population) will be on PD. Disappointingly very few haemodialysis patients choose or are prepared to dialyse at home ("home-haemo") which means that home haemodialysis accounts for only 2 % of the total RRT population. The split between CAPD and APD among those doing peritoneal dialysis is such that around one third choose CAPD and two thirds choose APD (Fig. 37.1).

Q3 How does haemodialysis work?

Haemodialysis was the first form of renal replacement therapy to be developed in the 1960s and remains the most common dialysis modality. Blood from the patient is pumped through a dialysis filter which removes waste products (urea) and fluid, before being returned to the patient. Urea moves from an area of high concentration to one of low concentration across a highly permeable dialysis membrane by a process known as diffusion. Fluid is removed by creating a negative transmembrane pressure in a process known as ultrafiltration. Successful haemodialysis requires good vascular access (see next question) (Fig. 37.2).

Q4   What is meant by the term vascular access?
Vascular access is the means by which patients are connected to their dialysis machines. Broadly speaking there are three types – fistulas, lines and grafts. An arteriovenous fistula is created by joining an artery to a vein in the wrist (radiocephalic fistula) or in the elbow (brachiocephalic fistula) under a local anaesthetic (Fig. 37.3). It is recommended that two thirds of patients should start haemodialysis with a fistula and that 80 % of all haemodialysis patients in each renal unit should have one. There are two types of line – temporary and tunnelled. Both are usually placed in the internal jugular vein under local anaesthetic.

Fig. 37.2 A basic haemodialysis circuit

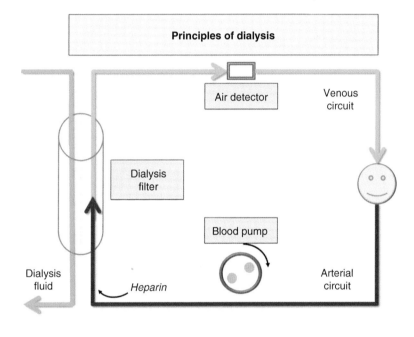

Fig. 37.3 An AV fistula sited in the forearm. Note blood leaving the arterial limb, passing through the dialyser and returning via the venous limb

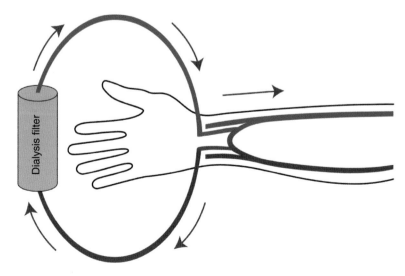

Temporary lines are fairly easy to insert and remove while tunnelled lines require considerably more expertise. The term 'tunnelled' refers to the subcutaneous tunnel leading to an exit site on the anterior chest wall which offers a greater degree of protection against infection than a temporary line. Grafts are the third form of access. They are created by joining arteries to veins by a short tube of Gore-tex. Currently less than 5 % of haemodialysis patients have one.

Q5 When should vascular access be discussed with patients?

The question of vascular access should be discussed once a patient with progressive renal failure has considered all the options and expressed a preference for haemodialysis rather than PD. This discussion will generally take place when eGFR is around 20 ml/min and will usually lead to referral for a fistula. A fistula is the preferred vascular access for haemodialysis because of the lower risk of clot formation and infection provided by the use of native vessels. Once a decision to create a fistula has been taken everything should be done to preserve the forearm veins by avoiding venepuncture and cannula insertion whenever possible.

Q6 Describe what happens when a fistula is created

Joining an artery to a vein in the wrist or antecubital fossa means that blood is diverted up the vein at arterial pressure without having to pass through the capillary network first. Exposing a vein to blood in this way leads to distension and thickening (so called arterialisation) of its wall. Fistulas take 6–8 weeks to mature and should be ready to use at the time of first dialysis which means the best time to create a fistula is at least 6–8 weeks before it is needed. Fistulas in people with diabetes and in non-diabetics with small arteries or difficult veins may need longer to mature. Timing is everything.

Q7 How do you know when to start dialysis in a patient with CKD?

The mnemonic AEIOU gives the five clinical indications for starting dialysis:

> **Box 37.1 Reasons for starting dialysis**
> **A** Acidosis eg if serum bicarbonate <10 mmol/l
> **E** Electrolytes eg when serum potassium >7 mmol/l
> **I** Inflammation i.e. pericarditis
> **O** Overload, meaning pulmonary oedema
> **U** Uraemia

The commonest reasons for starting dialysis are uraemia, fluid overload and hyperkalaemia. Uraemia, specifically "symptomatic uraemia", refers to patients who have a persistently high level of blood urea and develop the symptoms of anorexia, nausea and vomiting. Acidosis is rarely the main reason for starting dialysis but is often present when the patient becomes uraemic. Pericarditis is not present in every case, but is certainly an indication to start dialysis if the characteristic rub is heard. In practice we aim to start dialysis just before the symptoms or signs become clinically significant i.e. dialysis should be initiated to maintain wellbeing rather than to rescue from illness.

Q8 How does eGFR help us decide when to start dialysis?

Patients are monitored at the pre-dialysis clinic by estimating GFR using the MDRD equation. This is now reported routinely every time urea and electrolytes are requested. As a general rule preparation for dialysis should start in patients with progressive renal failure when they have CKD4 while dialysis should be considered when they have CKD5 and are beginning to develop symptoms. Knowing when to start dialysis is not always easy as some patients tolerate uraemia without symptoms for much longer than expected and eGFR may plateau at around 8–10 ml/min for months or even a year or so in others. The results of clinical trials suggest that with careful clinical management, dialysis may be delayed until either the eGFR drops below 7 ml/min or more traditional clinical indicators (see AEIOU above) for the initiation of dialysis are present.

Q9 Once a patient has started dialysis how do you know that he or she is being adequately dialysed?

Subjectively, patients should report that they start to feel better. Objectively, there are two main measures of dialysis adequacy in a haemodialysis patient. These are:

Box 37.2 Measures of dialysis adequacy
- Urea Reduction Ratio (URR).
- Kt/V.

The urea reduction ratio is calculated by subtracting the post dialysis urea from the pre-dialysis urea and dividing this by the pre-dialysis urea. A patient is considered to be adequately dialysed when his or her URR is >65 %. They would achieve this with a pre-dialysis urea of 24 mmol/l and a post dialysis urea of 8 mmol/l (24 − 8 ÷ 24=66 %). Kt/V is a measure of urea clearance corrected for total body water using a computer programme. Recommended weekly Kt/V for haemodialysis is a level >1.2.

Q10 List the complications of haemodialysis

These may be divided into patient, access and technical problems as shown in Box 37.3. We consider "crashing" on dialysis, hypertension and fluid overload in more detail in Chap. 40. Dysequilibrium syndrome occurs if urea is removed too rapidly from the bloodstream during the first dialysis, particularly in patients with chronic renal failure. Plasma osmolality falls and water moves into the brain. Clinical features include nausea, vomiting, headache, altered consciousness and rarely seizures. Dysequilibrium syndrome is much less common now than before because everyone is aware that it can happen and dialysis is usually initiated more gently than in the past. Some patients continue to experience nausea, vomiting and headache once established on dialysis, usually as a consequence of hypotension or dropping below their dry weight. Muscle cramps are another common and potentially troublesome problem, particularly towards the end of dialysis. For more detailed discussion of these and the other complications listed in Box 37.3,

see suggestion for further reading at end of this chapter,

Box 37.3 Complications of Dialysis

Patient Problems
Dialysis related hypotension – "crashing" on dialysis
Hypertension and fluid overload
Dysequilibrium Syndrome
Muscle cramps
Nausea and vomiting
Headache

Access Complications
Poor arterial flow rates
Recirculation
Infection
Thrombosis
Aneurysm formation

Technical Issues
Clotted circuit
Blood leak
Haemolysis
Air embolism
Dialyser reaction

Q11 You are asked to see a dialysis patient with ischaemic sounding chest pain. In what way does the diagnosis of acute coronary syndrome differ from that of a non-dialysis patient with acute coronary syndrome?

Acute coronary syndrome (ACS) in a dialysis patient is diagnosed when a patient with ischaemic sounding pain has sequential ECG changes and a 20 % or greater rise in troponin, as it is in patients who do not have kidney failure. Routine blood tests will include haemoglobin, which may well be low enough in CKD to have acted as a trigger for ischaemic pain (see Chap. 27). Serum troponin climbs following cardiac muscle damage and peaks at around 12 h. The main difference between those with and without renal disease is that troponin may be chronically elevated in dialysis patients who do not have acute coronary syndrome. Normal levels of troponin T are less than the 99th centile of the upper reference limit (<14 ng/l in our hospital) whereas in dialysis patients baseline levels of up to 200 ng/l have been recorded.

Q12   How does the management of acute coronary syndrome differ from that of a non-dialysis patient with acute coronary syndrome?

Dialysis patients presenting with ACS should be treated as in the nondialysis population with opiates for pain and antiplatelet drugs and low molecular weight heparin for ischaemia. The indications for coronary reperfusion by thrombolysis, percutaneous coronary intervention and CABG and for secondary prevention by statins and betablockers are the same. The only differences in management are that smaller doses of opiates and LMWH should be given. It is quite safe to use morphine once, but repeated doses will accumulate because of the renal failure, causing opioid toxicity. Dose reduction of LMWH for patients whose GFR is <30 ml/min is necessary because of the bleeding risk. This means, for example, giving dialysis patients with ACS enoxaparin 1 mg/kg subcutaneously once daily instead of 1 mg/kg SC twice daily.

Q13   A dialysis patient comes in for treatment on a Monday morning and says that he has been more short of breath overnight. What is the most likely explanation?

Pulmonary oedema. Dialysis patients may become breathless for all the reasons that a patient without kidney disease can become breathless, but breathlessness after a 3 day break from dialysis is almost always due to fluid overload. A raised JVP with bibasal crackles supports this diagnosis and a CXR usually confirms. Interdialytic weight gains that are consistently greater than 2 kg between dialyses are an important additional clue, as is a poor appetite for a week or two in a patient who comes in at the same weight (Fig. 37.4).

Q14   Describe the emergency management of a dialysis patient with pulmonary oedema.

This can be summarised in Box 37.4 below:

Box 37.4 Initial Management of Pulmonary Oedema in a Dialysis Patient
- Keep patient sitting up
- Give high flow oxygen to maintain SpO_2 94–98 %
- Morphine 5 mg IV with metoclopramide 5 mg IV to prevent nausea
- 2 puffs GTN Spray
- Isolated UF at a rate of 1,000 ml over 30 min initially

Remember to run the priming fluid off before connecting the patient up. After removing the first litre quickly, it is best to reduce the rate of

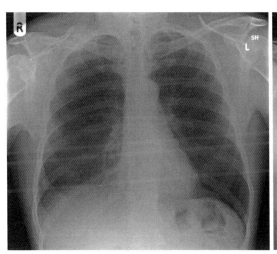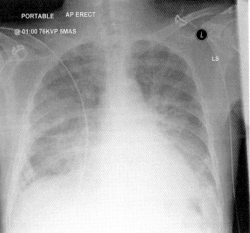

Fig. 37.4 Two chest X-rays showing the striking differences between normal lung fields (*right*) and pulmonary oedema (*left*)

fluid removal by ultrafiltration to a maximum of 500 ml per hour. UF rates greater than this are associated with a greater risk of symptomatic hypotension, and possibly also higher mortality. Note there is no role for frusemide in these circumstances as patients are highly unlikely to increase their urine output once they have become dialysis dependent, even if large doses of frusemide are given intravenously.

Q15   What would be the quickest way to get a breathless patient onto dialysis if he or she had no vascular access?

If you are inexperienced, the safest answer is a femoral line which can be inserted without having to lie the patient flat and which can be used without requiring a chest x-ray to confirm its position. By contrast, an experienced nephrologist might choose to insert an internal jugular line instead because the internal jugular vein will be hugely distended and the line very easy to put in with the patient in a semi-recumbent position under cover of morphine.

Q16   A dialysis patient has a URR that is persistently less than 60 %. What steps would you take to improve this?

There are four things you can do, as shown in Box 37.5:

> **Box 37.5 Actions Taken to Improve URR**
> 1. Increase the blood pump speed.
> 2. Use a bigger dialyser.
> 3. Increase the duration of dialysis.
> 4. Check that they are not recirculating.

Inadequate dialysis is a particular problem in patients with poor vascular access, in those who cannot tolerate a larger dialyser and when patients are not prepared to increase their dialysis times. Haemodialysis access recirculation occurs when dialysed blood returning through the venous needle re-enters the extracorporeal circuit through the arterial needle rather than returning to the systemic circulation, usually as a result of a venous stenosis (Fig. 37.5).

Q17   Dialysis adequacy means more than a URR >65 % or a Kt/V greater than 1.2. Discuss.

Optimal renal health means controlling fluid balance, potassium, acid base balance, blood pressure, renal bone disease and anaemia. It is important to address vascular, psychological and general health in addition, to assess for transplantation if this has not been done before and to consider dialysis withdrawal if and when this becomes appropriate. See Appendix 16 for more details.

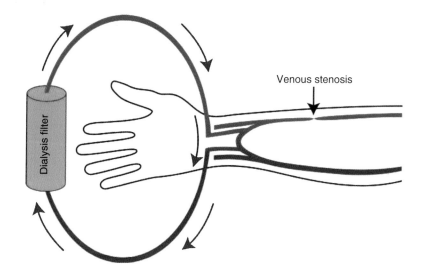

Fig. 37.5 Recirculation occurs when dialysed blood, returning to the patient via the venous needle, is re-circulated through the dialysis machine. This is usually due to a proximal venous stenosis (shown above)

37.1 Objectives: Haemodialysis

After reading this chapter, you should be able to answer the following:

Q1 Describe the different types of renal replacement therapy.

Q2 How many patients receiving RRT will be on haemodialysis, peritoneal dialysis or have a functioning transplant?

Q3 How does haemodialysis work?

Q4 What is meant by the term vascular access?

Q5 When should vascular access be discussed with patients?

Q6 Describe what happens when a fistula is created.

Q7 How do you know when to start dialysis in a patient with CKD?

Q8 How does eGFR help us decide when to start dialysis?

Q9 Once a patient has started dialysis how do you know that he or she is being adequately dialysed?

Q10 List the complications of haemodialysis

Q11 You are asked to see a dialysis patient with ischaemic sounding chest pain. In what way does the diagnosis of acute coronary syndrome differ from that of a non-dialysis patient with acute coronary syndrome?

Q12 How does the management of acute coronary syndrome differ from that of a non-dialysis patient with acute coronary syndrome?

Q13 A dialysis patient comes in for treatment on a Monday morning and says that he has been more short of breath overnight. What is the most likely explanation?

Q14 Describe the emergency management of a dialysis patient with pulmonary oedema.

Q15 What would be the quickest way to get a breathless patient onto dialysis if he or she had no vascular access?

Q16 A dialysis patient has a URR that is persistently less than 60 %. What steps would you take to improve this?

Q17 Dialysis adequacy means more than a URR >65 % or a Kt/V greater than 1.2. Discuss.

Further Reading

1. Mactier R, et al. Renal association clinical practice guidelines – haemodialysis. 2009. Access via www.renal.org.
2. Mujais SK, et al. Acute complications of haemodialysis and their prevention and treatment. In: Jacobs C et al., editors. Replacement of renal function by dialysis. Dordrecht: Springer Netherlands; 1996. p. 688–725.

Q1 What is PD and how does it differ from haemodialysis?

PD is a gentler form of renal replacement therapy than haemodialysis. Whereas an artificial membrane filters the blood in haemodialysis, peritoneal dialysis exploits the peritoneum as a natural semi-permeable membrane. It is usually performed by patients in their own homes. It involves running 2–2.5 litres of warmed dialysis fluid into the abdominal cavity using a thin rubber tube known as a Tenckhoff catheter, then waiting a few hours before draining the fluid out and infusing fresh fluid. This exchange of fluid takes around 20–30 min and is simple to learn. Most patients are competent after 2 days practice. The Tenckhoff catheter and the peritoneal membrane are to peritoneal dialysis, as vascular access and the artificial dialyser are to haemodialysis (Fig. 38.1).

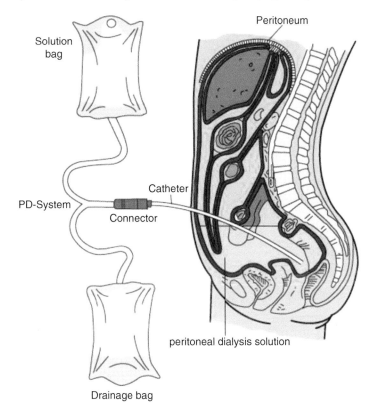

Fig. 38.1 Principles of peritoneal dialysis

Q2   How does peritoneal dialysis work?

In peritoneal dialysis, blood is filtered inside the body. Given the vast surface area and system of pores within the peritoneum, it acts as an ideal dialysis membrane. Blood is filtered through two mechanisms:

1. **Solute transport** – this is the movement of waste products (urea, creatinine and electrolytes) through simple diffusion down favourable concentration gradients. Dialysate contains balanced electrolyte solutions and lactate to correct acid-base disturbance.

2. **Ultrafiltration** – this is the movement of fluid out of peritoneal capillaries. It is driven by the osmotic gradient generated by the glucose-rich hyperosmotic dialysate.

Both processes are shown in the figure that follows. Most patients on CAPD will do 4 × 2 litre exchanges for solute removal with light (1.36 % glucose), medium (2.27 % glucose) or heavy (3.86 % glucose) bags for fluid removal. A patient with normal blood pressure and no oedema might be on 4 light bags. The more hypertensive and oedematous the patient the more benefit they will gain from medium and heavy bags (Fig. 38.2).

Q3   What is meant by the term CAPD?

Continuous ambulatory peritoneal dialysis (CAPD) is the term used to describe patients who run the PD fluid in and out themselves, and usually means four 2 litre exchanges each day. The timing of exchanges is not critical although patients usually do one when they get up in the morning, one at lunch time, one at teatime and one as they go to bed. This effectively gives them three 4–5 h dwells and one longer overnight dwell of 9–10 h (Fig. 38.3).

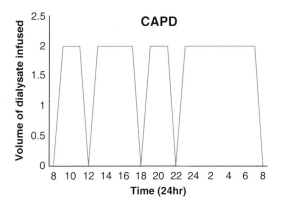

Fig. 38.3 CAPD exchanges demonstrating 3 day time exchanges and an overnight dwell

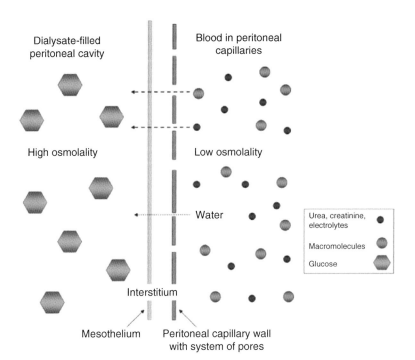

Fig. 38.2 Principles of solute transport and ultrafiltration across a semipermeable membrane

Q4   What is meant by the term APD?

Automated PD (APD) means programming a small bedside machine to exchange fluid automatically at night whilst the patient is asleep instead of undertaking manual exchanges of fluid through the day. CAPD and APD are interchangeable and some patients do both (Fig. 38.4).

Q5   Most patients choose APD rather than CAPD. Why?

The advantages to a patient of APD are as follows:
- APD gives the patient more daytime freedom.

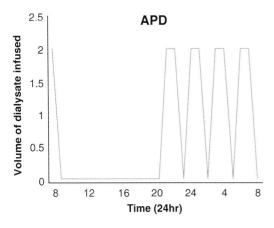

Fig. 38.4 APD. In this form of RRT, the patients have the option of being "dry" or "wet" during the day depending on whether further exchanges are required. The prescription above is for a patient who is dry during the day

- Less connections therefore less infection.
- More fluid and therefore more dialysis.
- Shorter dwell times and therefore better ultrafiltration.
- Less abdominal fullness because patient is supine during dialysis, therefore better appetite and less risk of hernia.

Q6   How do you judge whether a PD patient is adequately dialysed?

PD adequacy is judged on the following three parameters:
1. Clinical assessment – the well dialysed patient has a good appetite, no nausea, minimal fatigue and feels well.
2. Solute removal – we measure this by 24 h urine and PD fluid collection, together with a serum sample, to give total creatinine clearance in litres per week. Total creatinine clearance equals residual renal function plus peritoneal clearance. Current guidelines recommend a target of 50 litres per week for both CAPD and APD patients.
3. Fluid removal – patients should be both oedema free and normotensive.

Q7   List the complications of Peritoneal Dialysis.

The main complications are peritonitis, inadequate dialysis and loss of ultrafiltration. We discuss these in more detail below. The full list is summarised in Box 38.1

Box 38.1 Complications of Peritoneal Dialysis

Infection
Exit site and tunnel infection
Peritonitis
Failure
Inadequate dialysis
Loss of ultrafiltration
Encapsulating Peritoneal Sclerosis
Catheter related
Migration of catheter tip up out of pelvis – may be asymptomatic but often takes longer for fluid to drain in and out

Entrapment by omentum or adhesions – causing pain or obstruction to flow on infusion or drainage
Dialysate leaks and hernias
Leak from exit site
Leak through defect in diaphragm into pleural space – presents as a pleural effusion
Umbilical or incisional hernias – symptoms range from mild discomfort to intestinal obstruction

Q8   What should you do if a PD patient accidentally touches the end of their catheter or wakes up with the mini cap off?

The patient should attend their local Renal Unit for prophylactic antibiotic. Add 1 g vancomycin to a 2 litre bag of physioneal 1.36 % (light) CAPD fluid, allow to dwell for 6 h then drain. Alternatively, if the roller clamp on catheter has not been opened and no fluid has been run in, the extension set may be changed by a PD nurse.

Q9   What should you do if a PD patient phones in with abdominal pain?

> **PD & abdominal pain? → Assume peritonitis until proven otherwise.**

Ask the patient to drain out to see if cloudy and then bring the fluid up to the Renal Unit, or ask the patient to come up to the Renal Unit and then witness them doing an exchange. If they have no fluid in they should do an exchange with a 2 h dwell. This is the only way to confirm or exclude a cloudy bag if a patient has difficulty in distinguishing cloudy from clear fluid, which many do.

Q10   What should you do if a PD patient presents with a cloudy bag?

The likely diagnosis is peritonitis. The patient should come up to the Renal Unit with their cloudy bag which must be sent as an emergency to microbiology requesting gram stain, white cell count and culture. You should examine their exit site and tunnel, and swab this if it looks infected, plus send a nasal swab. Thereafter you should follow the flow chart on investigation and management of suspected PD peritonitis (Appendix 17).

Q11   Which organisms are most commonly responsible for PD peritonitis?

The variety and frequency with which different organisms are isolated are as follows:

> **Box 38.2 Organisms Commonly Responsible for PD Peritonitis**
> - **Gram positive organisms** cause up to 75 % of all cases. Staph. epidermidis infections are usually mild and cured with appropriate antibiotic therapy. Staph aureus is associated with a much more severe picture often leading to loss of the catheter and also with a significant risk of death.
> - **Gram negative organisms** account for around 20 % of all cases. Pseudomonas infections are the most dangerous. They are difficult to eradicate and lead to loss of the peritoneal cavity.
> - **Fungal peritonitis** is uncommon, is generally caused by candida species and requires catheter removal.
> - **Mixed gram positive and gram negative** infections often result from bowel perforation and carry a bad prognosis.
> - **Culture negative peritonitis** accounts for around 10 % of all cases. These may be due to coagulase negative staphylococci that are difficult to grow or to chemical irritants in the dialysis fluid or may occur because the patient has inadvertently used antibiotics before culture.

Q12   What antibiotics are normally recommend for PD peritonitis?

Vancomycin to cover gram positive organisms and ceftazidime to cover gram negative organisms. For doses, see flow chart on investigation and management of suspected PD peritonitis (Appendix 17). Gentamicin has gone out of favour because of the risk of deafness, vertigo and loss of residual renal function.

Q13   A PD patient has a total creatinine clearance of less than 50 litres per week. What steps would you take to improve this?

This result suggests inadequate dialysis. You can increase solute removal by prescribing more fluid e.g. 2.5 litre bags four times daily (10 litres per day) instead of 2 litres four times daily (8 litres). Alternatively, and because many patients do not tolerate a 2.5 litre fill volume, you could switch the patient from CAPD to APD and increase the volume of dialysis fluid by adding a day dwell or a daytime exchange.

Q14 A PD patient presents with moderate oedema. What steps can you take to improve ultrafiltration?

Increase the concentration of glucose in the dialysis fluid in order to create an osmotic gradient. Medium bags contain 2.27 % glucose and heavy bags 3.86 % glucose. The higher the osmotic gradient generated by a higher glucose concentration the greater the fluid drawn across the peritoneal membrane. It goes without saying that in order to achieve an osmotic gradient blood glucose must be lower than PD fluid glucose (Fig. 38.5).

For hypertensive and oedematous patients there is also the option of using icodextrin (Extraneal), a glucose polymer capable of creating an osmotic pressure gradient without all the drawbacks of glucose (see below). Icodextrin is only suitable for long dwells e.g. overnight, and has no place in the management of patients who require rapid fluid removal.

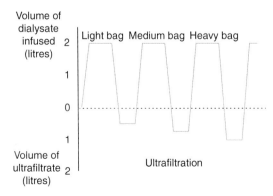

Fig. 38.5 Effects of light, medium and heavy bags on ultrafiltration

Q15 What should you do if a PD patient presents with gross fluid overload?

Under these circumstances there is little option but to admit for APD using 3.86 % fluid or a combination of 3.86 and 2.27 %. Advice should always be sought from those experienced in PD. Ideally the patient should have 3 × 5 litre bags and 16 h of treatment. If the patient is diabetic then he or she will require an insulin infusion in order to keep the blood glucose between 7 and 11 mmol/l – otherwise there will be no osmotic gradient.

Q16 Why is it best to limit the use of medium and heavy bags in peritoneal dialysis?

The glucose load in medium and heavy bags can create problems for diabetic patients particularly if their blood glucose is poorly controlled, may contribute to obesity and may also be a risk factor for Encapsulating Peritoneal Sclerosis.

Q17 What do you know about Encapsulating Peritoneal Sclerosis (EPS)?

EPS is an important and often fatal complication of PD, characterised by progressive 'encapsulation' of bowel loops that leads to bowel obstruction and severe malnutrition. Risk factors include duration of PD, recurrent peritonitis and exposure of the peritoneal membrane to high concentrations of glucose. Diagnosis is usually confirmed by CT scan. There is as yet no specific treatment for EPS. Aggressive nutritional support is advised. Steroids have been used for anti-inflammatory and tamoxifen for antifibrotic effects. Surgery for intestinal obstruction can be life-saving in selected cases

Q18 What should you do if a PD patient leaks fluid from their exit site or develops lower abdominal subcutaneous swelling?

An exit site leak will be quite obvious. Lower abdominal subcutaneous swelling usually means that they are leaking fluid from the peritoneal entry site. There may well be genital oedema too. The patient should come up to the Renal Unit for review. An exit site leak is usually managed by giving 1 g of vancomycin IV over 1 h. The correct action for both types of leak is then to drain out and rest the peritoneum for a period that may vary from 3 or 4 days to 3 or 4 weeks depending on the severity of the leak. Depending on their serum potassium, fluid balance and blood urea they may or may not require temporary haemodialysis. Sometimes it is possible to continue low volume PD using the APD machine with the patient supine.

38.1 Objectives: Peritoneal Dialysis

After reading this chapter, you should be able to answer the following:

Q1 What is PD and how does it differ from haemodialysis?

Q2 How does peritoneal dialysis work?

Q3 What is meant by the term CAPD?

Q4 What is meant by the term APD?

Q5 Most patients choose APD rather than CAPD. Why?

Q6 How do you judge whether a PD patient is adequately dialysed?

Q7 List the complications of Peritoneal Dialysis.

Q8 What should you do if a PD patient accidentally touches the end of their catheter or wakes up with the mini cap off?

Q9 What should you do if a PD patient phones in with abdominal pain?

Q10 What should you do if a PD patient presents with a cloudy bag?

Q11 Which organisms are most commonly responsible for PD peritonitis?

Q12 What antibiotics are normally recommend for PD peritonitis?

Q13 A PD patient has a total creatinine clearance of less than 50 litres per week. What steps would you take to improve this?

Q14 A PD patient presents with moderate oedema. What steps can you take to improve ultrafiltration?

Q15 What should you do if a PD patient presents with gross fluid overload?

Q16 Why is it best to limit the use of medium and heavy bags in peritoneal dialysis?

Q17 What do you know about Encapsulating Peritoneal Sclerosis (EPS)?

Q18 What should you do if a PD patient leaks fluid from their exit site or develops lower abdominal subcutaneous swelling?

Further Reading

1. Woodrow G, Davies S. Renal association clinical practice guidelines – peritoneal dialysis. Access via www.renal.org.

Q1 When should a patient be considered for a renal transplant?

Renal transplants have been shown to improve survival and quality of life in patients who are under 75 years of age. This is not to say that patients over 75 will not benefit, simply that no evidence exists of a survival advantage. Older patients are certainly at more risk of having a heart attack or stroke at the time of their surgery or shortly afterwards. Risks and benefits should be considered carefully in all age groups.

Q2 What different types of renal transplant are there?

Cadaveric transplantation remains most common and still accounts for around two thirds of all transplants, though living donor transplantation is increasing. Simultaneous pancreas-kidney transplants are a treatment option for patients with kidney failure and type 1 (but not type 2) diabetes. Pre-emptive transplantation means receiving a kidney before starting dialysis. Altruistic donation is the giving of a kidney from a living person to a friend or to a stranger. The different types of transplant are summarised in Fig. 39.1

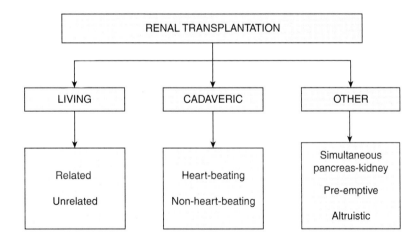

Fig. 39.1 Categories of renal transplantation

Q3   What is meant by donation after brain death (DBD)?

Donation after brain death is also known as heart beating kidney donation. The typical donor is a patient with a significant brain injury requiring life support by ventilation in whom brain stem death has been confirmed by the following criteria:

Box 39.1 Criteria for Brain Stem Death
- No pupil reflexes.
- No corneal reflex.
- No nystagmus when ice cold water is run into each ear.
- No response to painful stimulus.
- No gag reflex.
- No attempt to breathe unaided when the ventilator is switched off and the $PaCO_2$ is allowed to rise over 6.5 kPa at a time when the patient continues to receive oxygen.

The incidence of brain stem death is declining year on year due to tighter road safety regulations. In clinical practice the brain stem death tests are conducted by two doctors on two separate occasions usually 10 or 15 min apart. Neither doctor should have anything to do with the transplantation. Sedatives should be withdrawn for 24 h before conducting brain stem death tests. Once brain stem death has been established, the patient is taken to theatre and the kidneys are removed while the heart is still beating, before complications occur. Complications of brain stem death include hypotension, diabetes insipidus, DIC and arrhythmia.

Q4   What is meant by donation after cardiac death (DCD)?

Donation after cardiac death is also known as non-heart beating kidney donation. This is an altogether more difficult area. The doctors looking after the patient, who will invariably be in the intensive care unit, need to separate discussion about futility from discussion about organ donation. There is then a 2 h window after stopping therapy during which retrieval of a viable kidney is possible, provided the patient dies during that time. Not all patients in whom active treatment is withdrawn will die and not all of those who do die will do so within 2 h.

Q5   How is consent obtained from the relatives?

In the UK the relatives still have the right of veto even if the patient has carried a donor card. In order to donate a kidney, the family must 'opt in'. Many doctors believe more kidneys would be donated if patients were asked to 'opt out' instead ie it is assumed they will donate their kidneys unless they have specifically signed a register to say they will not do so. For the time being the opt-in system remains in place in the UK.

Q6   How are cadaveric organs allocated?

By blood group and tissue typing. Donors and recipients should be blood group and tissue type compatible. The four blood groups are A, B, AB and O and the way in which the matching works is as follows:

Box 39.2 ABO Compatibilities
- A can receive from A or O.
- B can receive from B or O.
- AB can receive from anybody.
- O can only receive from O.

Patients are also tissue typed by their HLA (Human Leukocyte Antigen) antigens. We use three of these for tissue typing: the A, B and DR antigens. Each of us has 2 A, 2 B and 2 DR antigens, one from each parent. The best tissue matches are A, B and DR identical. This is referred to as an OOO mismatch. Mismatches for the A and B antigens are not as important as mismatches on the DR antigen. Fewer mismatches allow for a lower dose of immunosuppressant drugs and a lower risk of acute rejection. In addition, a better match lowers the risk that the patient will develop antibodies to the donor antigens (donor specific antibodies) – a phenomenon which could increase the chances of rejection and also make future transplants more difficult.

Q7   What written information is a transplant surgeon likely to give a patient before adding their name to the waiting list?

Having established that the patient is likely to benefit from a renal transplant the surgeon will explain that the waiting time can be 3–4 years if the patient has to wait for a cadaveric transplant. He/she will then discuss surgery and how the kidney is placed superficially in the left or right iliac fossa with blood vessels plumbed into the iliac vessels and the donor ureter into the recipient bladder. There will be a ureteric stent at the time of surgery and this will remain in place for approximately 6 weeks in order to hold the ureteric surgical suture line open until it has fully healed (Fig. 39.2).

Patients can expect to be in hospital for at least a week and in some cases several weeks depending on how long the transplant kidney takes to work. Living kidneys usually start to work immediately but a cadaveric kidney can take several days or even weeks (Fig. 39.3). Patients will be told that at least 90 % of grafts will be working at 1 year, and that 50 % will still be working at 10 and 15-years following cadaveric and living donor kidney transplants respectively.

The reasons for failure of a transplant will also be discussed. Less than 1 % of kidneys will never work and a similar number will fail early on due to blood clot. The surgeon will discuss the mech-

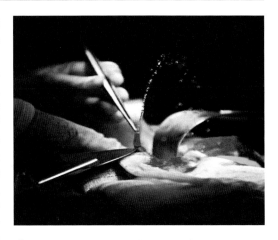

Fig. 39.3 Intra-operative urine production

anisms of rejection and how repeated episodes of rejection can damage the kidney. It will also be mentioned that some of the medication used to prevent rejection, particularly ciclosporin and tacrolimus, can in the long term fur up the small blood vessels within the kidney and cause it to fail. Patients must accept these risks before proceeding to transplantation.

Q8   Name the immunosuppressive drugs that are commonly used to prevent rejection?

> **Box 39.3 Commonly Used Immuosuppresive Drugs**
> - Prednisolone.
> - Mycophenolate mofetil/ azathioprine
> - Tacrolimus/ciclosporin

Nearly all patients will receive initial triple therapy with prednisolone, mycophenolate and tacrolimus. Mycophenolate is an anti-proliferative drug and tacrolimus a calcineurin inhibitor (CNI). They are more potent, more modern and more expensive than their predecessors azathioprine and ciclosporin respectively. Occasionally a dose reduction or drug switch to one of the less common immunosuppressant drugs is necessary if a patient develops an unacceptable drug side effect (eg switch to sirolimus in a patient with recurrent skin malignancy).

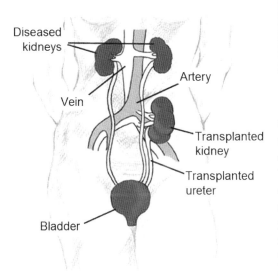

Fig. 39.2 Placement of renal transplant

Q9   Discuss the side effects of the immuno-suppressive drugs.

The main risk is that of infection, not only in the perioperative period, but for the duration of immunosuppression ie the life of the transplant (see Q11 below). There are in addition some drug specific side effects (Box 39.4).

Box 39.4 Side Effects of Immunosuppressive Drugs

Prednisolone
Obesity, diabetes, hypertension, osteoporosis, peptic ulceration

Azathioprine
Neutropenia, skin rash and malignancy.

Mycophenolate
Diarrhoea, myelotoxicity.

Ciclosporin
Nephrotoxicity, gum hypertrophy, hirsutism, hypertension.

Tacrolimus
Diabetes and tremor are more likely, nephrotoxicity as likely, and gum hypertrophy and hirsutism less likely than ciclosporin. Tremor can be particularly troublesome when serum levels are at the upper end of the therapeutic range.

In practice the most troublesome side effects are weight gain with steroids, diarrhoea with mycophenolate, neutropenia with azathioprine and nephrotoxicity with both ciclosporin and tacrolimus. Concerns about steroid side effects have led some centres to develop steroid free or minimisation protocols.

Q10   A patient whose transplant has been functioning well with a baseline creatinine of 106 μmol/L comes to the clinic where it is found that his creatinine has doubled. What could account for this?

Patients with a transplant can experience all the usual causes of AKI (see elsewhere) but are more likely to have a cause that is directly related to their transplant.

- Rejection
- Ciclosporin or tacrolimus toxicity
- Infection

- Obstruction
- Transplant artery stenosis
- Recurrence of the original disease

The approach to such a problem is fairly straightforward. A patient in whom the creatinine has risen more than you would expect should have an urgent repeat sample followed by transplant ultrasound, urine culture and ciclosporin/tacrolimus level if the raised creatinine is confirmed. If these tests do not give the answer then they must be referred for a transplant biopsy. Two types of rejection are recognised: cell mediated and vascular. Vascular rejection is often antibody mediated and usually more aggressive. Focal segmental glomerulosclerosis and IgA nephropathy both have a tendency to recur in a transplant.

Q11   Apart from graft failure what other risks should a patient be aware of?

The three big risks are opportunistic infections, vascular disease and cancer. All three are related at least in part to the use of immunosuppressive drugs. The most important opportunistic organisms in a transplant patient are cytomegalovirus (CMV), varicella zoster virus (VZV) and pneumocystis pneumonia (PCP). Renal transplant recipients have a lower risk of cardiovascular disease than those who remain on dialysis, though the risk is still higher than in the general population. Immunosuppressant medication can worsen hypertension, lipid profiles and increase the risk of diabetes, all contributing to cardiovascular disease which is a leading cause of death in transplant patients. Cancers are also more common as a result of immunosuppression. Most cancers are only slightly commoner than in the general population, though skin cancers, lymphomas and cervical cancers pose special risks.

Q12   What type of illness does CMV cause and how may this be treated?

CMV infection can cause graft dysfunction as well as a systemic illness characterised by swinging fever, deranged liver function tests and leucopenia. The most serious manifestation is pneumonitis but fortunately this is now rare. The best test for CMV infection is a CMV PCR. Treatment is reserved for serious infection and should be with either oral valgancyclovir or intravenous ganciclovir for 14 days adjusted according to renal function (see manufacturer's instructions). Tissue-invasive disease may require 4–6 weeks therapy.

Q13 Can CMV infection be prevented?

Yes, though what is done depends on the CMV status of donor and recipient. In the box below D stands for donor, R for recipient, (–) for CMV negative and (+) for CMV positive.

Box 39.5 Prophylaxis Advice for CMV

D (–) R(–) No prophylaxis required.

D (+) R(–) Give prophylaxis with val-ganciclovir for 200 days immediately post-transplantation according to estimated GFR: 900 mg od if eGFR >60 ml/min; 450 mg od if eGFR 40–59 ml/min; 450 mg alternate days if eGFR 25–39 ml/min; 450 mg once weekly if eGFR 10–24 ml/min; do not use if eGFR <10 ml/min.

D (+/–) R (+) Prophylaxis for 200 days if heavily immunosuppressed ie for patients receiving induction immunosuppression with OKT3 or ATG.

Q14 When should pneumocystis pneumonia be suspected and how can this be diagnosed and treated?

Pneumocystis jirovecii is the organism responsible for the opportunistic infection pneumocystis pneumonia (PCP) which should be suspected in transplant patients with fever and breathlessness, with or without dry cough. Chest x-ray usually shows patchy interstitial infiltrates but lobar patterns have also been described. Taking a patient for a walk to demonstrate exercise induced hypoxia may be useful in cases where the chest x-ray is unremarkable. Diagnosis is by visualisation of the organism in induced sputum, bronchial lavage fluid or tissue from transbronchial biopsy. Treatment is with intravenous Septrin as guided by the microbiologists.

Q15 Can pneumocystis pneumonia be prevented?

All transplant patients receive Septrin 480 mg once daily for 6 months immediately post transplantation in order to reduce their risk of pneumocystis pneumonia.

Q16 Discuss what can happen and what you might do if a susceptible transplant patient became infected with VZV.

Fulminant VZV can occur in susceptible patients i.e. those with no antibodies to the VZ virus, if they are exposed to patients with chickenpox or herpes zoster. The incubation period is up to 21 days of the initial contact. Affected patient then present with a typical skin rash which may become haemorrhagic and be associated with pneumonia leading to multi-organ failure. Prophylaxis is with varicella zoster immune globulin (VZIG) which should be administered within 7 days of contact with chickenpox or herpes zoster. Treatment is with intravenous acyclovir. The following case report shows just how serious VZV infection may be in a susceptible transplant patient.

Case Report

A 30 year old male renal transplant recipient with a diagnosis of Wegener's granulomatosis contacted the Renal Unit within 24 h of exposure to a family member with zoster. He attended the Accident and Emergency Unit where he received VZIG 1 g intramuscularly. Four weeks later he presented with a maculopapular rash on his head, neck and upper body. The following day he developed mouth ulceration and the rash became vesicular. Varicella was diagnosed and he was given intravenous acyclovir 10 mg/kg every 8 h. Over the next 24 h his condition deteriorated rapidly with bleeding from venepuncture sites, spontaneous bruising and acute kidney injury. He died of multi-organ failure within 60 h of admission. A stored serum sample, prior to receiving VZIG, showed no antibodies to VZV.

Robertson S et al. Fulminating varicella despite prophylactic immune globulin and intravenous acyclovir in a renal transplant recipient: should renal patients be vaccinated against VZV before transplantation? *Clinical Transplantation* 2005; 20: 136–138; with permission from John Wiley and sons.

Q17   What steps can be taken to reduce the risk of VZV infection in a transplant patient?

Between 1 and 2 % of the patients awaiting a transplant in the UK will be susceptible to VZV. Testing for VZV antibody should be a routine part of the transplant workup and VZV susceptible patients should be offered VZV vaccine. This is a live vaccine which must be given 3 months before transplantation in order to reduce the risk of fulminating varicella after the transplant. Patients who are already on the waiting list for transplant should be suspended temporarily from the list after vaccination.

Q18   What should you do with immunosuppressive therapy when a transplant patient develops a severe infection?

When a transplant patient develops a severe infection whether this be due to CMV, pneumocystis or to some other cause, then it is best to stop their anti-proliferative medicaiton (azathioprine/ mycophenolate), and consider either continuing or stopping their calcineurin inhibitor (ciclosporin/tacrolimus) depending on the severity of infection, while continuing steroids alone as hydrocortisone IV in the acute phase. Patients on long term low-dose steroid should have the dose increased to cover the acute illness and reduced in convalescence. There is a theoretical risk the kidney might reject but in practice this hardly ever happens and anyway it would be better to have a live patient on dialysis than a dead one as a result of pneumonia. As the patient recovers from their illness, reintroduce immunosuppression at a lower dose eg prednisolone and tacrolimus rather than prednisolone, mycophenolate and tacrolimus.

Q19   Is it ever safe to vaccinate a patient with a functioning transplant?

Live vaccines including mumps, measles, rubella and varicella zoster should be avoided in immunosuppressed patients. Inactivated vaccines eg influenza and pneumococcus are generally safe for transplant patients but should not be given during acute illnesses.

Q20   How likely is a renal transplant patient to develop cancer?

One third of the UK population will develop cancer at some point in their lives. Cancer is commoner in transplant patients as a result of immunosuppression, such that 25 % of patients who live for 20 years after a transplant will develop some type of cancer. Skin cancers, lymphoma, cervical cancer and colorectal cancer all occur more commonly than in the general population. There is no increased risk of breast cancer

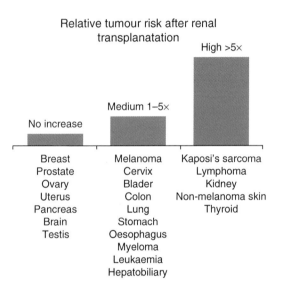

Fig. 39.4 Relative tumour risk after renal transplantation (Reproduced from Clinical Practice Guidelines. Postoperative Care of the Kidney Transplant Recipient. UK Renal Association, 2011)

or prostate cancer. Relative risks of these and other cancers are shown in Fig. 39.4.

Q21   Which skin cancers occur in transplant patients?

Skin cancers account for 95 % of all malignancy in transplant patients. Basal cell carcinoma (BCC) is commoner than squamous cell carcinoma (SCC) in the general population, whereas in patients who receive a transplant SCC occurs more commonly than BCC. Melanoma is also more common in transplant patients. Risk factors for SCC and BCC include older age at transplantation, duration of immunosuppression, male sex, increased UV exposure, cigarette smoking and the presence of actinic keratoses.

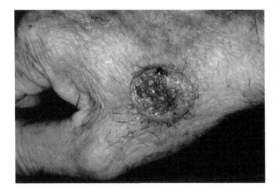

Fig. 39.5 Large basal cell carcinoma

Prevention is better than cure. Patients should be advised to avoid sun burning and deliberate tanning by avoiding sun between 11 am and 3 pm and by using sunblock creams. All patients must be offered annual skin checks (Fig. 39.5).

Q22 What type of lymphomas may occur in transplant patients?

Lymphoma occurs in 1–2 % of transplant patients usually within 1 year of the transplant. 96 % are non Hodgkin's lymphomas. Post transplant lymphoproliferative disorder (PTLD) is a unique form of lymphoma driven by exposure to EB virus (see Fig. 39.6) and fuelled by immunosuppressive drug therapy. Treatment consists of reducing the dose of immunosuppressive drugs. Some patients also require rituximab, a monoclonal antibody directed against B cells, as was the case in the report that follows.

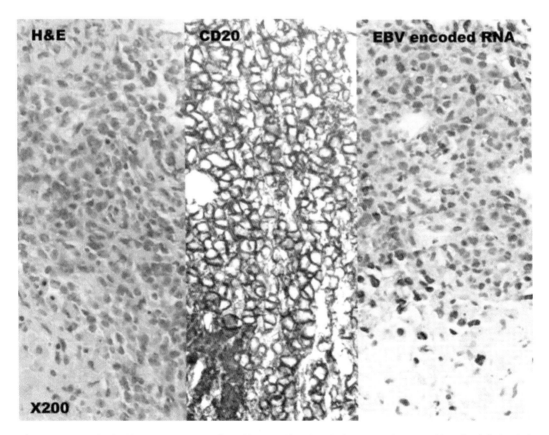

Fig. 39.6 The cells in this tumour were confirmed immunohistochemically as lymphocytes of B cell origin by their CD20 positivity and were also strongly positive for EBV encoded RNA

Case Report

A 38 year old woman presented with a glandular fever like illness and positive EBV serology, 16 months after a second cadaveric transplant. Her underlying diagnosis was focal segmental glomerulosclerosis, an early recurrence of which had led to the loss of her first graft. Her second transplant was perfectly matched but highly sensitised so she had been given basiliximab as induction therapy followed by prednisolone, tacrolimus and mycophenolate. Imaging showed a 6 cm soft tissue mass inferior to the transplanted kidney, encircling the femoral vessels. There were no other sites involved. A diagnosis of high grade non-Hodgkin's lymphoma was made by biopsy. The cells in this tumour were strongly positive for EBV encoded RNA (see figure). Withdrawal of tacrolimus and mycophenolate followed by infusion of rituximab led to a significant reduction in tumour size. When seen at the clinic 6 years after her initial presentation with PTLD serum creatinine was 137 µmol/l. She was taking prednisolone 5 mg daily only for immunosuppression. Her lymphoma was no longer visible on ultrasound.

Image reproduced with permission from Selvarajah V et al. Post-transplant lymphoproliferative disorder: case report and review of susceptibility to EBV in the Scottish adult renal transplant pool. *NDT Plus* 2009; 2: 52–54; with permission from Oxford University Press

39.1   Objectives: Renal Transplantation

After reading this chapter, you should be able to answer the following:

Q1   When should a patient be considered for a renal transplant?

Q2   What different types of renal transplant are there?

Q3   What is meant by donation after brain death (DBD)?

Q4   What is meant by donation after cardiac death (DCD)?

Q5   How is consent obtained from the relatives?

Q6   How are cadaveric organs allocated?

Q7   What written information is a transplant surgeon likely to give a patient before adding their name to the waiting list?

Q8   Name the immunosuppressive drugs that are commonly used to prevent rejection?

Q9   Name the side effects of the immunosuppressive drugs.

Q10   A patient whose transplant has been functioning well with a creatinine of 106 µmol/L comes to the clinic where it is found that his creatinine has doubled. What could account for this?

Q11   Apart from graft failure what other risks should a patient be aware of?

Q12   What type of illness does CMV cause and how may this be treated?

Q13   Can CMV infection be prevented?

Q14   When should pneumocystis pneumonia be suspected and how can this be diagnosed and treated?

Q15   Can pneumocystis pneumonia be prevented?

Q16   Discuss what can happen and what you might do if a susceptible transplant patient became infected with VZV.

Q17 What steps can be taken to reduce the risk of VZV infection in a transplant patient?

Q18 What should you do with immunosuppressive therapy when a transplant patient develops a severe infection?

Q19 Is it ever safe to vaccinate a patient with a functioning transplant?

Q20 How likely is a renal transplant patient to develop cancer?

Q21 Which skin cancers occur in transplant patients?

Q22 What type of lymphomas may occur in transplant patients?

Further Reading

1. British Transplant Society Guidelines. Available at http://www.bts.org.uk/BTS/Guidelines_Standards/Current/BTS/Guidelines_Standards/Current_Guidelines.aspx.
2. Renal Association Clinical Practice Guideline for Post-operative care of the kidney transplant recipient, 2011. Available at http://www.renal.org/guidelines/modules/post-operative-care-of-the-kidney-transplant-recipient.

Q1   The majority of haemodialysis patients are hypertensive. Why?

There are likely to be two reasons. First, they may be hypertensive because the disease that was responsible for their kidney failure was associated with or caused hypertension. This is true for patients with hypertensive nephrosclerosis, and for most patients with glomerulonephritis, diabetic nephropathy and polycystic kidney disease. Second, they may be hypertensive because they are overloaded. A direct relation between volume status and blood pressure is well recognised in dialysis patients. The higher the interdialytic weight gain, the greater the pre-dialysis blood pressure and the greater is the decrease in blood pressure during dialysis.

Q2   What is the relation between blood pressure and mortality in dialysis patients and how does this differ from that seen in the general population?

BP and mortality are inversely related in dialysis patients, which is the opposite that in the general population (Fig. 40.1). The likely explanation is that cardiac disease in haemodialysis patients lowers blood pressure and raises mortality (not that lowering blood pressure in renal patients is harmful).

Q3   What are the targets for pre and post dialysis blood pressures?

Expert opinion, which is based on observational data rather than randomised trials, suggests a pre-dialysis SBP 140–160 mmHg and a pre-dialysis DBP between 70 and 90 mmHg. Optimal post dialysis BP is thought to be 135–155 mmHg for systolic and unchanged at 70–90 mmHg for diastolic. Patients with fistulas may be feeling apprehensive about the insertion of their dialysis needles, and if so this could exaggerate the alarm reaction that occurs every time a patient's blood pressure is taken. For this reason, the first blood pressure reading after a patient has started dialysis, which is usually within 5 min of initiating treatment before any significant fluid has been removed, may give a better indication of pre-dialysis blood pressure.

Q4   What is the key therapeutic goal for the hypertensive haemodialysis patient?

Normovolaemia. This can usually be achieved by salt restriction, ultrafiltration and by reducing dialysate sodium concentration, provided the patient is willing to play their part by limiting

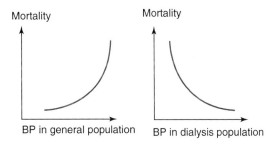

Fig. 40.1 Relationship between mortality and BP in general and dialysis population

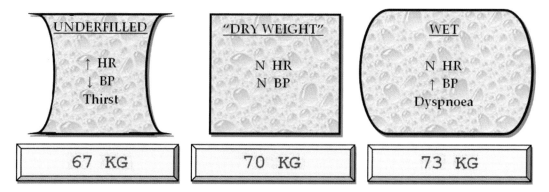

Fig. 40.2 Clinical pointers to fluid status in a dialysis patient

weight gains between dialysis. Reduction of dry weight is worth attempting in a hypertensive dialysis patient even in the absence of clinical signs of volume overload. If successful then this can reduce and sometimes eliminate the need for antihypertensive drugs. For these reasons it is always more logical to re-evaluate dry weight than to start or increase antihypertensive drugs.

Q5   What does the term dry weight mean?

"Dry weight" is the term used to indicate a dialysis patient's optimal body weight. This is the weight at which they are euvolaemic, i.e. neither too wet nor too dry. A common issue for patients on long term RRT is fluid overload or being "wet", especially if unfortunate enough to be anuric. Bearing in mind that 1 kg of body weight approximates 1 litre of water a patient's weight can be used to monitor their fluid balance, and in particular their inter-dialytic weight gain (see Q8) (Fig. 40.2).

Q6   How might you know if a patient was over their dry weight?

Practically, by checking their weight pre-dialysis. Clinically, a patient who is over their dry weight will usually have oedema and/or be breathless, though a surprising number of overloaded patients have no symptoms whatsoever. They might well be hypertensive. The most likely reason for being over dry weight in a dialysis dependent patient is failure to adhere to fluid restriction.

Q7   What other causes of peripheral oedema may occur in a dialysis patient?

Other causes of peripheral oedema in a dialysis patient include the nephrotic syndrome, heart failure, deep vein thrombosis, cellulitis and a ruptured Baker's cyst. The commonest drugs causing oedema are the dihydropyridine calcium channel blockers, such as amlodipine or nifedipine. Oedema is usually an acceptable price to pay for the benefit of being on these drugs and is not a reason to discontinue the calcium blocker unless the oedema is very marked or distressing.

Q8   What advice should a dialysis patient be given in order to reduce his or her risk of becoming overloaded?

For some patients, particularly if they are thirsty, fluid restriction is the hardest part of dialysis. Measuring fluid intake – which could become an all-consuming task – is not recommended. Instead, patients should be advised to limit their interdialytic weight gain to a maximum of 2 kg, which is equivalent to 2 litres of fluid. They should be reminded that fluids include soups, puddings, jellies and ice cream in addition to cups of tea, coffee or water. For patients who do not pass any urine at all, fluid restriction of this order can be quite demanding. As a rough guide an anuric patient should be advised to drink not more than 800 ml per day.

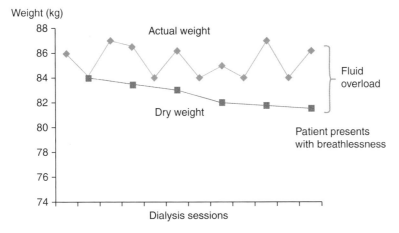

Fig. 40.3 Weight on dialysis. The "actual weight" line shows the rapid changes in weight experienced by dialysis patients due to loss/gain of fluid. Observing the "dry weight" line (the patient's ideal weight) we can see that as time passes they are losing weight (protein/fat). If this goes unnoticed, we may falsely believe that at 86 kg, they are only carrying an extra 2 litres, as opposed to true value of 4 litres extra. This can results in symptomatic overload – shown here as a presentation with breathlessness

Q9   Can a patient whose pre-dialysis weight is not greater than expected still be overloaded?

Yes. This usually means that the patient's dry weight has dropped because they have not been eating properly. This should prompt questions about appetite and food intake, and should always lead to referral to the renal dietitian. You should check dialysis adequacy as poor URR may be the cause of poor appetite and food intake (Fig. 40.3).

Q10   What might happen to the patient if you take too much fluid off too quickly?

The patient will usually complain of dizziness and feeling warm or sick, just before they 'crash' or may just crash without any preceding symptoms. 'Crash' is the term used to describe a patient who collapses suddenly on dialysis as a result of excessive fluid removal. This can be a frightening experience for the patient, the nurses and the other patients in the unit. It is the equivalent of a very bad faint. The patient will be hypotensive, is likely to be bradycardic and may fit. In severe cases it can look as if they have had a cardiac arrest.

Q11   What precisely should you do when a patient crashes?

Move quickly to tip the patient backwards, stop ultrafiltration and administer saline and oxygen. The volume of saline required will vary from patient to patient. You should run in at least 250 ml stat then review progress. Give oxygen by facial mask at 10 litres per minute. Screen the patient off if possible and reassure the other patients.

Q12   What steps can you take to ensure that a patient does not crash during dialysis?

You can reduce the risk of crashing by making a careful assessment of the fluid that must be removed at the beginning of dialysis and by using the online blood volume monitor. The ultrafiltration rate should not normally exceed 500 ml per hour. The online blood volume monitor measures a patient's haematocrit which is the proportion of the blood volume that is occupied by their red blood cells. If fluid is removed too rapidly from the blood compartment and is not replaced by fluid from the tissues then the haematocrit will rise. If the haematocrit rises too far or too quickly then the patient is likely to crash.

Q13 **If it is not possible to control a dialysis patient's blood pressure by removing fluid then which antihypertensive drugs can you use?**

The short answer is that all classes of antihypertensive drugs may be used to treat hypertension in haemodialysis patients, with one or two provisos. Dihydropyridine calcium channel blockers eg amlodipine are probably the easiest to use although their commonest side effect is ankle swelling which may make it more difficult to assess dry weight. The pros and cons of the other antihypertensive drugs in dialysis patients are shown in Box 40.1.

Box 40.1 Pros and Cons of Antihypertensive Agents

ACE inhibitors
Commonest side effect is cough. Not advised if pre-dialysis potassium >5.0 mmol/l.

Angiotensin receptor blockers
Generally well tolerated. Not advised if pre-dialysis potassium >5.0 mmol/l.

α-blockers
Often makes patients feel non-specifically unwell. Not contraindicated in advanced renal failure.

β-blockers
Commonly cause cold hands and lethargy. Not contraindicated in advanced renal failure.

Calcium channel blockers
Main side effect is oedema but otherwise well tolerated. Not contraindicated in advanced renal failure.

Thiazides
Unlikely to be effective when serum creatinine >150 μmol/l.

Spironolactone
Not advised if pre-dialysis potassium >4.5 mmol/l.

Loop diuretic
Little point in using unless overloaded and able to mount a diuresis. May require a larger dose up to 500 mg daily because of advanced renal failure.

Q14 **Antihypertensive drugs may increase the risk of symptomatic intradialytic hypotension. Why?**

By interfering with the compensatory vasoconstriction that maintains BP in the face of the rapid reduction in intravascular volume that occurs during haemodialysis. It is for this reason that we often advise a hypertensive patient who is taking antihypertensive drugs to withhold these until after his or her dialysis session has been completed.

40.1   Objectives: Hypertension and Fluid Balance in Dialysis Patients

Q1 The majority of haemodialysis patients are hypertensive. Why?

Q2 What is the relation between blood pressure and mortality in dialysis patients and how does this differ from that seen in the general population?

Q3 What are the targets for pre and post dialysis blood pressures?

Q4 What is the key therapeutic goal for the hypertensive haemodialysis patient?

Q5 What does the term dry weight mean?

Q6 How might you know if a patient was over their dry weight?

Q7 What other causes of peripheral oedema may occur in a dialysis patient?

Q8 What advice should a dialysis patient be given in order to reduce his or her risk of becoming overloaded?

Q9 Can a patient whose pre-dialysis weight is not greater than expected still be overloaded?

Q10 What might happen to the patient if you take too much fluid off too quickly?

Q11 What precisely should you do when a patient crashes?

Q12 What steps can you take to ensure that a patient does not crash during dialysis?

Q13 If it is not possible to control a dialysis patient's blood pressure by removing fluid then which antihypertensive drugs can you use?

Q14 Antihypertensive drugs may increase the risk of symptomatic intradialytic hypotension. Why?

Q1   Describe the different types of vascular access for haemodialysis

There are four, summarised in Box 41.1. Fistulas are the preferred form of vascular access as discussed in Chap. 37.

Box 41.1 Different Types of Vascular Access

1. Arterio-Venous Fistula (usually known as a fistula)
2. Arterio-Venous Graft (usually known as a graft)
3. Tunnelled Central Venous Catheter (usually known as a tunnelled line)
4. Non-Tunnelled Central Venous Catheter (usually known as a temporary line)

Q2   Why do some patients dialyse with a tunnelled line?

Tunnelled lines are an effective and very quick method of achieving vascular access but are more likely to become infected than fistulas. Other complications of tunnelled lines include central venous stenosis and poor flow due to kinking or formation of a fibrin sheath on the outside of the catheter. Despite these limitations some patients dialyse quite successfully with a tunnelled line rather than a fistula. Indications for a tunnelled line are shown in the box:

Box 41.2 Common Reasons for Long-Term Central Venous Catheter Use

Late presenters in whom there has not been time to create a fistula.

- Patients with poor peripheral vessels in whom a fistula is not technically possible.
- Patients with chronic heart failure whose cardiac output might be further compromised by a fistula, because so much of it goes through the fistula.
- Patients with hypotension whose blood pressure might be further lowered by a fistula.
- Very elderly patients (>80 years) who may have poor peripheral vessels, chronic heart failure, hypotension and poor life expectancy in whom a fistula might not be of any real benefit.
- Rarely, patients with a true needle phobia will refuse a fistula or a graft

---

Q3   What is the best vein for a tunnelled line and why?

The right internal jugular vein is preferred for catheter placement due to its direct continuity with the superior vena cava and the right atrium. Alternative sites are the left internal jugular vein (more difficult to place and 50 % risk of venous stenosis), subclavian vein (should be avoided

M. Findlay, C. Isles, *Clinical Companion in Nephrology*,
DOI 10.1007/978-3-319-14868-7_41, © Springer International Publishing Switzerland 2015

because of higher incidence of central venous stenosis) and femoral vein (higher risk of infection).

Q4   What is the correct position for a tunnelled line?

For an internal jugular line the catheter tip should be positioned in the mid right atrium to optimise flow (Fig. 41.1). Be aware that the catheter tip may retract by as much as 1–2 cm when the patient adopts an upright position as the chest wall is pulled downwards particularly in obese patients or women with large breasts. An internal jugular catheter whose tip lies in the lower right atrium may come in contact with the tricuspid valve and so cause dysrhythmias. When the femoral vein is used for haemodialysis, the length of the catheter must be 20 cm or more and the catheter tip should be positioned in the common iliac vein or inferior vena cava. When the tip of a shorter catheter is positioned in the external iliac vein, high rates of recirculation will be encountered.

Q5   What can be done to minimise the risk of infection with tunnelled lines?

Some units may give prophylactic flucloxacillin or vancomycin at the time of insertion but this is not a universal recommendation. We no longer recommend dressings but lock our lines with a taurolodine (antimicrobial) and citrate (anticoagulant) solution called Taurolock and screen our patients for staphylococcal nasal carriage. Up to half of all dialysis patients are nasal carriers of staph aureus. Nasal mupirocin eradicates staph aureus and has been shown to reduce the incidence of staphylococcal catheter related septicaemia fourfold. Because of this all staph aureus nasal carriers with tunnelled lines should receive mupirocin three times daily to both nostrils for 7 days. The evidence for and against these measures is summarised below. We consider catheter related bloodstream infection in more detail in Chap. 42 (Table 41.1).

Q6   How do you take blood from a tunnelled line?

Ideally this should only be done by renal unit staff. If you have to use a tunnelled line in an emergency then you must do so aseptically with gloves, mask and dressing pack. Remember to

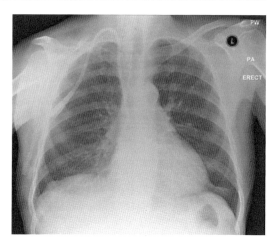

Fig. 41.1   The correct position of a tunnelled line

Table 41.1   Methods used to reduce catheter related infection

Method	Efficacy
Prophylactic antibiotics at time of insertion	No benefit, may encourage resistant organisms
Occlusive dressings	No evidence of benefit
Antiseptic line locks	Taurolock effective
Elimination of staphylococcal nasal carriage	Nasal mupirocin effective

aspirate the first 2 ml containing the taurolodine/citrate solution and discard before drawing blood for analysis. Remember also to replace the line lock when you have finished.

Q7   What should you look for when you examine a tunnelled line exit site?

The exit site should be examined for signs of inflammation or tunnel track infections eg erythema, pain, secretions, crusts or abscess formation. You should also record whether the dacron cuff is visible. If so then the catheter will usually require to be replaced. For more information on line related infection, see Chap. 42.

Q8   What is an acceptable blood flow rate for a tunnelled catheter?

Catheters generally allow a blood flow up to 350 ml/min which is necessary for adequate dialysis. Longer catheters provide less blood flow compared to shorter catheters of the same diameter which is a problem particularly for femoral vein catheters. Catheter flow rates of less than 200 ml/min at any site suggests blockage or partial blockage.

Q9 What might be done for a tunnelled line with blood flow rate less than 200 ml/min?

Steps that might be taken to improve tunnelled line flow rates are shown in the box.

Box 41.3 Stepwise Protocol for Maintaining Central Line Patency

If the line is placed in the internal jugular and less than 2 weeks old, check the position of the catheter tip by chest x-ray.

- Follow the urokinase protocol for blocked tunnelled lines (see Appendix 18).
- If patency cannot be restored then a contrast study should be arranged to show whether poor flow is due to intraluminal thrombus, catheter tip thrombus or fibrin sheath.
- A fibrin sheath surrounding the catheter tip requires the prolonged infusion of urokinase to dissolve the clot. If this is not successful then the sheath may be stripped by means of a snare catheter, inserted through the femoral vein. This is probably worth trying but is not always successful.
- Persisting catheter dysfunction requires a new catheter. This can be done over a guidewire unless a fibrin sheath is the cause of the problem, as the fibrin sheath will simply encase the new catheter. For this reason the insertion of a new catheter at a new venous site may be the better option.

41.1 Objectives: Tunnelled Dialysis Catheters

After reading this chapter, you should be able to answer the following:

Q1 Describe the different types of vascular access for haemodialysis.

Q2 Why do some patients dialyse with a tunnelled line?

Q3 What is the best vein for a tunnelled catheter and why?

Q4 What is the correct position for a tunnelled line?

Q5 What can be done to minimise the risk of infection with tunnelled lines?

Q6 How do you take blood from a tunnelled line?

Q7 What should you look for when you examine a tunnelled line exit site?

Q8 What is an acceptable blood flow rate for a tunnelled catheter?

Q9 What might be done for a tunnelled line with blood flow rate less than 200 ml/min?

Further Reading

1. Fluck R, Kumwenda M. Vascular access for haemodialysis. Clinical Practice Guidelines, 5th edition. UK Renal Association, 2011. Access via www.renal.org/guidelines/modules/vascular-access-for-haemodialysis.

Catheter Related Blood Stream Infection

Q1 How common is catheter related blood stream infection (CRBSI)?

Catheter related blood stream infection (CRBSI) is the most important complication of central venous dialysis catheters. The risk of tunnelled line bacteraemia is around 1–3 episodes per 1,000 catheter days in most renal units. Tunnelled lines have lower rates of infection than temporary lines and jugular placement carries a lower risk than femoral. Bacteraemia is approximately ten times more common with lines than with fistulas and this is one of the reasons why a fistula is the preferred form of vascular access for haemodialysis. Tunnelled lines are also associated with significantly higher risks of death from infection than fistulas and grafts.

Q2 When should you suspect CRBSI?

This diagnosis must be considered in all dialysis patients with a central venous catheter (CVC) who present with pyrexia or acutely raised inflammatory markers. Patients with CRBSI will classically present between dialyses with a rigor and a temperature of 39°. However, the presentation can be subtle and have only minor signs such as low grade fever, hypothermia, hypotension, loss of glycaemic control, lethargy and confusion. Less commonly patients will present with disseminated infection (e.g. discitis) from an untreated access infection.

Q3 How should you investigate a patient with suspected CRBSI?

Promptly, by simultaneous culture of blood from the line and the periphery before commencing antibiotic therapy. Blood culture from the line should be from the catheter hub after first removing the line lock i.e. you should discard about 3 ml before using a separate syringe for the culture. Clinical examination is usually unrevealing, which is often a pointer to the catheter as the source of infection (i.e. absence of other sources of infection). The exit site and/or tunnel are not always inflamed. Alternative sources of infection should be considered with a focussed history, examination, imaging (especially chest x-ray) and laboratory testing (urine culture if possible). You should also remember to check white cell count and CRP, and swab both the exit site and nose.

Q4 What are the likely infecting organisms in a patient with CRBSI?

The great majority are staphylococci (Fig. 42.1). Coagulase negative staphylococci are usually regarded as skin contaminants when grown from peripheral blood cultures but may be pathogenic if isolated from a dialysis line or any patients with indwelling prosthetic material.

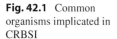

Fig. 42.1 Common organisms implicated in CRBSI

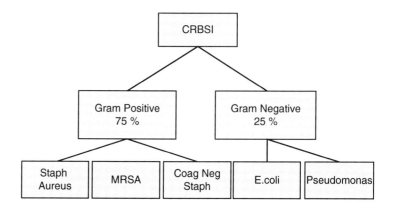

Q5 What antibiotic or antibiotics would you choose to give while waiting for the result of the blood culture?

In general antibiotics that can be given post dialysis (vancomycin, teicoplanin, cefazolin and ceftazidime) are preferred. Vancomycin is the first choice for empirical therapy of gram positive organisms in settings where MRSA is prevalent while teicoplanin is a suitable alternative if there has been a previous allergic reaction to vancomycin. Some units give a single dose of gentamicin in view of its rapid bactericidal effect but longer courses are not advised unless the results of blood culture show that gentamicin is the only option. It is difficult to achieve safe trough levels with post dialysis gentamicin, thereby increasing the risk of ototoxicity and loss of residual renal function. If it is felt necessary to provide continuing gram negative cover, e.g. patient looks very unwell, then ceftazidime is first choice. Ciprofloxacin can be given as an alternative to ceftazidime to a patient who is only moderately unwell as it has high oral bioavailability.

Q6 How might your choice of antibiotic change after the results of blood culture become available?

If flucloxacillin sensitive staph aureus is grown on culture then best advice is to switch from vancomycin (bacteriostatic) to flucloxacillin (bactericidal). In practice the advantages of vancomycin, which can be given through the line at the end of dialysis and which only needs

to be given on dialysis days, outweigh those of flucloxacillin, for which a suitable vein requires to be found four times daily. An option favoured by many units is to continue vancomycin while adding oral rifampicin to augment its anti-staphylococcal activity. Vancomycin dose should be adjusted to take account of residual renal function and the type of dialysis e.g. high flux, haemodiafiltration, daily dialysis, using trough levels (Box 42.1). All renal units will have agreed protocols for CRBSI. For more detailed discussion of this topic see the European Best Practice Guideline (referenced below)

Box 42.1 Recommended Antibiotics for CRBSI

Initial dose vancomycin:	based on body weight: 1G if 40–59 kg, 1.5G if 60–90 kg, 2.0G if >90 kg
Subsequent dose vancomycin:	to maintain trough level 15–20 mg/L
Initial dose gentamicin:	2.5 mg/kg up to max 180 mg
Subsequent doses gentamicin:	not advised
Ceftazidime:	500 mg – 1G every 24–48 h
Loading dose teicoplanin:	400 mg every 12 h for three doses
Subsequent doses teicoplanin:	200–400 mg every 48–72 h

Q7 Should tunnelled lines always be removed?

This is not always necessary. Patients with uncomplicated CRBSI and those in whom catheter removal would result in complete loss of vascular access may be treated by leaving the catheter in situ and giving IV antibiotics for 3 weeks with antibiotic lock. This approach may cure over two thirds of uncomplicated infections. All other patients should have their tunnelled lines removed. The European Best Practice Guidelines recommend an antibiotic lock as part of the treatment of CRBSI though each unit will have its own protocol and local practice may vary. If an antibiotic lock is used then it will likely contain gentamicin which does not precipitate when diluted with heparin and which has both gram negative and anti-staphylococcal activity. Those with staph aureus and MRSA septicaemias should have transoesophageal echo routinely to exclude endocarditis before making a decision on whether the duration of antibiotics should be for 3 or 6 weeks (Fig. 42.2).

Q8 How would your management differ if the patient had a temporary line?

Temporary line septicaemia should never be treated by leaving the catheter in situ or with antibiotic locks. Fortunately, and unlike tunnelled lines which are secured with a dacron cuff, temporary lines slip out very easily. The line should be removed as soon as CRBSI is suspected, ie usually following a rigor with temperature 39° and without waiting for the blood culture to go positive. This is done with the patient in the head down position and should be followed by pressure over the exit site for 5 min, or until haemostasis is achieved, and an air occlusive dressing i.e. Tegaderm. Remember to send the catheter tip for culture. Ideally the patient should remain "plastic free" for as long as possible whilst continuing antibiotic treatment to reduce re-infection, before inserting a new line.

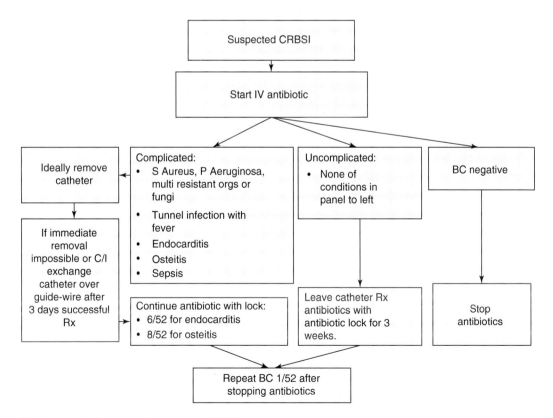

Fig. 42.2 Stepwise approach to suspected CRBSI

42.1   Objectives: Catheter Related Blood Stream Infection

After reading this chapter, you should be able to answer the following:

Q1 How common is catheter related blood stream infection (CRBSI)?

Q2 When should you suspect CRBSI?

Q3 How should you investigate a patient with suspected CRBSI?

Q4 What are the likely infecting organisms in a patient with CRBSI?

Q5 What antibiotic or antibiotics would you choose to give while waiting for the result of the blood culture?

Q6 How might your choice of antibiotic change after the results of blood culture become available?

Q7 Should tunnelled lines always be removed?

Q8 How would your management differ if the patient had a temporary line?

Further Reading

1. Vanholder R, et al. Diagnosis, prevention and treatment of haemodialysis catheter-related bloodstream infections (CRBSI): a position statement of European Renal Best Practice (ERBP). NDT Plus. 2010;3(3): 234–46.

**Q1 Describe the treatment options for
elderly patients.**

In theory all patients with established renal
failure have the option of hospital haemodialysis,
home haemodialysis, peritoneal dialysis, transplantation or conservative care (Fig. 43.1). In
practice, no Scottish patients over the age of
80 years are currently being treated by home haemodialysis. There is no theoretical reason why an
elderly renal patient should not have a pre-emptive transplant though this also does not happen.
If a trial of renal replacement therapy is chosen,
this effectively means a choice between hospital
based haemodialysis and peritoneal dialysis at
home. Studies suggest that with appropriate mul-
tidisciplinary support, over 50 % of an elderly
population eligible for PD will choose this form
of treatment. However, the uptake is much lower.
A UK Renal Registry analysis of patients under
65 years on 31/12/2012 showed that 63 % had a
functioning transplant, 31 % were treated by haemodialysis, and only 6 % were undergoing PD. In
the over 65s the proportion with a functioning
transplant dropped to 27 % with most of the
remaining patients receiving haemodialysis
(64 %) rather than PD (9 %).

**Q2 When should you consider conservative
care as a treatment option?**

We believe conservative care is an important treatment option for all patients over

80 years of age and that it may also be the correct decision for younger patients if they are
frail or have multiple comorbid illnesses. This
is not to say that patients over 80 years of age
cannot dialyse successfully, but to recognise
that patients aren't obliged to dialyse if after
careful consideration of the pros and cons they
choose not to. Frailty and comorbidity occur
more commonly in the elderly, and for many
frail, comorbid elderly patients renal replacement therapy may just prove to be too
demanding.

**Q3 How well does serum creatinine predict
the need for dialysis in the elderly?**

Less well than in a younger person. For a
given level of serum creatinine, GFR will always
be lower in the elderly, especially if underweight.
In these circumstances the Cockcroft Gault equation may well give a more precise estimate of
residual function than the MDRD formula

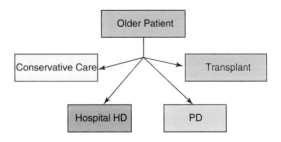

Fig. 43.1 Treatment modalities for older patients

M. Findlay, C. Isles, *Clinical Companion in Nephrology*,
DOI 10.1007/978-3-319-14868-7_43, © Springer International Publishing Switzerland 2015

(because the Cockcroft Gault takes body weight into account). For example, an 80 year old woman who has a serum creatinine of 300 umol/l and weighs 50 kg will have a creatinine clearance of 10 ml/min. By contrast a 50 year old man with the same level of creatinine who weighs 80 kg will have a clearance of 30 ml/min. The elderly underweight woman has end stage kidney disease while her younger male counterpart clearly does not.

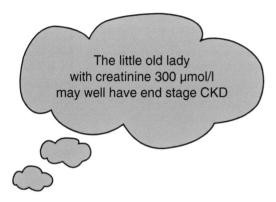

The little old lady with creatinine 300 μmol/l may well have end stage CKD

Q4 Why do more elderly patients choose hospital haemodialysis than PD?

It is likely that physical problems, social circumstances and cognitive impairment conspire to make PD less attractive in the elderly. This is ironic given that in a recent UK study scores estimating the intrusion of therapy and quality of life were found to be better in PD patients than in those who received haemodialysis. Some units may promote PD more than others as judged by a fourfold variation in uptake between units reported to the UK Renal Registry in 2012.

Q5 How might the uptake of PD be increased in the elderly?

A recent development has been assisted automated PD. Automated PD allows the patient to be treated at night with a portable machine that pumps fluid in and out of their peritoneal cavity automatically. With assisted APD a fully trained healthcare assistant visits daily – emptying drainage bags, checking drained fluid for cloudiness, setting up the machine for the next treatment, inspecting the catheter exit site and reviewing stocks of treatment fluids and drugs. These assis-

tants maintain contact with the parent unit which intervenes if problems arise.

Q6 By how much does dialysis increase survival in the elderly?

A recent report from the Lister Unit in the UK revisited the survival of elderly CKD patients in a non-randomised study. Eighty-two percent were treated by RRT while 18 % received conservative management. Survival was calculated from the first recorded eGFR of <15 ml/min rather than from the onset of dialysis, and adjusted for comorbidity. The survival advantage associated with dialysis fell to 4 months when subjects aged 75 years were analysed separately (Fig. 43.2). The take home message from this paper was that elderly patients who receive renal replacement therapy are only likely to achieve a worthwhile survival advantage if they have low co-morbidity.

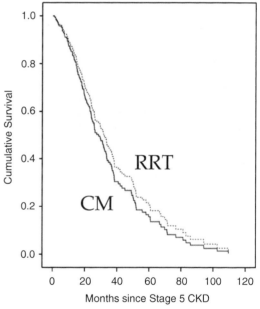

Fig. 43.2 Survival curves of patients aged >75 years who were managed conservatively (*CM*) or by renal replacement therapy (*RRT*) adjusted for age, gender, ethnicity, diabetes and comorbidity. Survival advantage in RRT patients was less than 4 months, which was not statistically significant (Reproduced with permission from Chandna et al. Survival of elderly patients with stage 5 CKD: comparison of conservative management and renal replacement therapy. *NDT* 2011;26:1608–14; Oxford University Press)

Q7   Elderly dialysis patients are susceptible to most of the so called 'Geriatric Giants'. Discuss.

The 'Geriatric Giants' are infection, immobility, instability, incontinence and intellectual impairment. In CKD stage 5, infection is an ever present increased risk, particularly with tunnelled lines, whilst immobility is common as demonstrated by the number of patients who attend dialysis in wheelchairs. Instability leads to falls and these are greatly increased in chronic kidney disease. Urinary incontinence may be a lesser problem than in the general population since many dialysis patients pass little or no urine. Impaired intellect occurs in 10–15 % of patients with an eGFR of <30 ml/min and when it does so it adds to the burden of a very demanding form of treatment.

Q8   What kind of quality life can an elderly dialysis patient expect?

Physical quality of life is generally lower in elderly RRT patients than in age matched populations who do not have chronic kidney disease. In contrast, the emotional quality of life in elderly RRT patients is usually as good as that of their peers in the general population. A recent US study followed the progress of all patients 80 years or older who started dialysis between 2000 and 2005. At the start of renal replacement therapy, 78 % were living independently at home, 15 % were living at home with assistance and 6 % were already in nursing homes. After 2 years of follow up only 11 % of the original cohort (18 % of those still alive) were still living independently at home. The remainder required community or private care support or had been transferred to a nursing home.

Q9   In what way is renal palliative care similar to that of non-renal palliative care?

The four key principles are exactly the same. These are that:
1. Informative, timely and sensitive communication is an essential component of each individual patient's care
2. Significant decisions about a patient's care, including diagnosing dying, are made on the basis of multi-disciplinary discussion

3. Each individual patient's physical, psychological, social and spiritual needs are recognised and addressed as far as is possible
4. Consideration is given to the wellbeing of relatives or carers attending the patient

Q10   In what way does renal palliative care differ from non-renal palliative care?

Renal palliative care for elderly dialysis patients should begin at the time of diagnosis and continue throughout life. It differs from non-renal palliative care in many respects, not least of which are the management of renal anaemia and pain. Treatment of symptomatic anaemia with ESAs and intravenous iron, one of the renal success stories of the last decade, can improve wellbeing while reducing the need for blood transfusion. Pain is a frequent symptom in patients with end stage CKD and pain control is often challenging (see also Chap. 33). The active metabolites of morphine accumulate in renal failure and may cause severe symptoms (myoclonic jerks, profound narcosis and respiratory depression) before relieving pain. It is preferable therefore, to use opiates that do not accumulate in renal disease such as fentanyl or alfentanil. Detailed advice including drug doses is given in the Renal Palliative Care guideline referenced at the end of this chapter but in practice a fentanyl patch, with oxycodone orally for breakthrough pain at home or alfentanil subcutaneously in hospital, is usually effective (Fig. 43.3). Patients whose pain is not controlled should be referred to the palliative care team if this has not been done already. Renal patients also have an option denied to the rest of us of dialysis withdrawal, which effectively allows them to die at the time of their choosing.

Q11   How commonly do elderly renal patients choose to withdraw from dialysis?

Dialysis withdrawal is now the commonest cause of death for elderly patients on renal replacement therapy. Twenty percent of all deaths in a recent French study were due to dialysis withdrawal which was defined as death occurring more than 3 days after the last dialysis. Average survival time after the last treatment session was

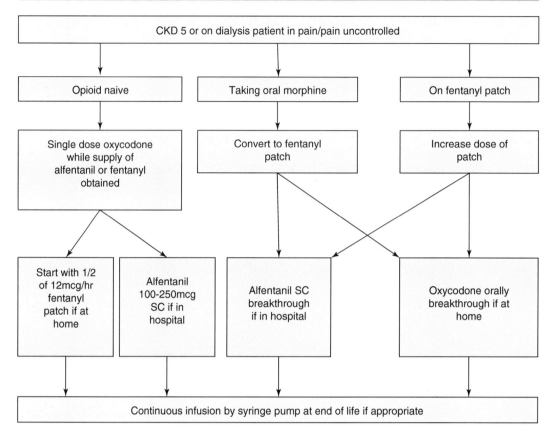

Fig. 43.3 Pain management in CKD 5, on dialysis and at end of life

8.5 days. Survival is likely to be longer in patients with residual renal function. Discussion of dialysis withdrawal can be a very sensitive issue if it is seen as the withholding of a lifesaving treatment in an elderly patient. Many elderly dialysis patients perceive their quality of life to be much better than we might surmise and nephrologists need to accept that, though it may not be what we would wish for ourselves, some patients appear content to continue dialysis three times a week in hospital to enable them to be at home not doing very much but surrounded by their families.

Q12 How do renal patients die?

The trajectory for organ systems failure is shown in Fig. 43.4. The gradual decline in function punctuated by hospital admissions which become more frequent towards the end of life is common in renal failure. Death often seems 'sudden' to many relatives of renal patients even if the gradual and progressive decline in the patient's health has been obvious to the hospital team. Most patients whose dialysis is withdrawn die after becoming progressively more drowsy and slipping into uraemic coma. If death occurs suddenly, asystole due to hyperkalaemia is the likely cause. Pain, myoclonus, dyspnoea, respiratory tract secretions and nausea should be anticipated by prescribing alfentanil, midazolam, hyoscine butylbromide and levomepromazine SC as required. Continuous infusion by syringe pumps may be indicated for each of these drugs if symptoms persist. Many renal units now have renal palliative care nurse specialists who are skilled in uraemic symptom control and whose remit also includes support for the family and carers, both before and after death.

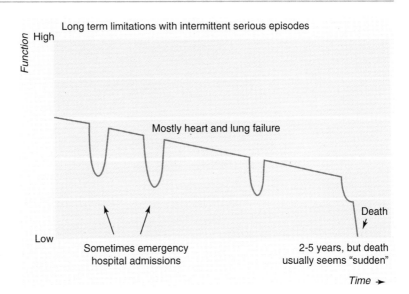

Fig. 43.4 Stepwise deterioration leading to death observed in frail patients (Reproduced from Murray S et al. Illness trajectories and palliative care. *BMJ* 2005;330:1077–11 with permission from BMJ Publishing Group Ltd)

43.1 Objectives: The Challenges of Renal Replacement Therapy in the Elderly

Q1 Describe the treatment options for elderly patients.

Q2 When should you consider conservative care as a treatment option?

Q3 How well does serum creatinine predict the need for dialysis in the elderly?

Q4 Why do more elderly patients choose hospital haemodialysis than PD?

Q5 How might the uptake of PD be increased in the elderly?

Q6 By how much does dialysis increase survival in the elderly?

Q7 Elderly dialysis patients are susceptible to most of the so called 'Geriatric Giants'. Discuss.

Q8 What kind of quality life can an elderly dialysis patient expect?

Q9 In what way is renal palliative care similar to that of non-renal palliative care?

Q10 In what way does renal palliative care differ from non renal palliative care?

Q11 How commonly do elderly renal patients choose to withdraw from dialysis?

Q12 How do renal patients die?

Further Reading

1. Chandna SM, et al. Survival of elderly patients with stage 5 CKD: comparison of conservative management and renal replacement therapy. Nephrol Dial Transplant. 2011;26:1608–14.
2. Renal Palliative Care. www.palliativecareguidelines. scot.nhs.uk/documentys/RenalLastDays.pdf.
3. The Renal Association. UK Renal Registry. The Sixteenth Annual Report. 2013. www.renalreg.org.

Appendices

Appendix 1 Treatment of Hyponatraemia

Severity	Action
Hyponatraemia with severe symptoms	1. First hour management, regardless of whether hyponatraemia is acute or chronic, give intravenous infusion of 150 mL 3 % hypertonic saline or equivalent over 20 min
	2. Check serum sodium after 20 min while repeating an infusion of 150 mL 3 % hypertonic saline or equivalent over the next 20 min
	3. Repeat (1) and (2) twice or until a target of 5 mmol/L increase in serum sodium concentration is achieved
	4. Manage patients with severely symptomatic hyponatraemia in medical HDU
Hyponatraemia with moderately severe symptoms	1. Treat the cause wherever possible, stopping medications and other factors that can contribute to or provoke the hyponatraemia
	2. Immediate treatment with a single intravenous infusion of 150 mL 3 % hypertonic saline or equivalent over 20 min aiming for a 5 mmol/L/24 h increase in serum sodium
	3. Aim to limit increase in serum sodium to 10 mmol/L in the first 24 h and 8 mmol/L during every 24 h thereafter, until a serum sodium of 130 mmol/L is reached
	4. Check serum sodium after 1, 6 and 12 h
	5. Consider other causes for the symptoms if they do not improve with an increase in serum sodium
	6. Manage patient as in severely symptomatic hyponatraemia if the serum sodium further decreases despite treating the underlying diagnosis
Acute hyponatraemia without severe or moderately severe symptoms	1. If possible, stop fluids, medications and other factors that can contribute to or provoke the hyponatraemia
	2. If the acute decrease in serum sodium is >10 mmol/L, give a single intravenous infusion of 150 mL 3 % hypertonic saline or equivalent over 20 min
	3. Check the serum sodium after 4 h

M. Findlay, C. Isles, *Clinical Companion in Nephrology,*
DOI 10.1007/978-3-319-14868-7, © Springer International Publishing Switzerland 2015

Severity	Action
Chronic hyponatraemia without severe or moderately severe symptoms	1. Stop non-essential fluids, medications and other factors that can contribute to or provoke the hyponatraemia
	2. In mild hyponatraemia (Na 130–135 mmol/l), there is no need to treat with the sole aim of increasing the serum sodium
	3. In moderate (Na 125–129 mmol/l) or profound (<125 mmol/l) hyponatraemia, aim to avoid an increase in serum sodium >10 mmol/L during the first 24 h and >8 mmol/L during every 24 h thereafter
	4. Patients with reduced circulating volume – infuse saline 0.9 % 6–8 hourly. Note that in case of haemodynamic instability, the need for rapid fluid resuscitation overrides the risk of an overly rapid increase in serum sodium concentration
	5. Patients with expanded extracellular fluid – restrict fluid to prevent further fluid overload. May require salt and fluid restriction with loop diuretic if fluid restriction alone fails
	6. Patients with SIADH – restrict fluid intake as first-line treatment in moderate or profound hyponatraemia. Give combination of low dose loop diuretics and oral sodium chloride if fluid restriction alone fails. Lithium, demeclocycline and vasopressin receptor antagonists no longer recommended

Further Reading

1. Spasovski G, et al. Clinical practice guideline on diagnosis and treatment of hyponatraemia. Eur J Endocrinol. 2014;170:G1–47.

Appendix 2 Treatment of Hypokalaemia

Severity	Action
Mild **3.0–3.5 mmol/l**	1. Approx deficit 200–300 mmol K
	2. Give around 60–80 mmol K per day orally as Slow K 2 tabs four times daily (64 mmol K) or Sando K 2 tabs three times daily (72 mmol K)
	3. Or try potassium preservation with e.g. amiloride 5 mg daily or ACEI/ARB – useful if hypokalaemia is diuretic induced, hypertensive or heart failure
	4. Check U&E twice weekly
Moderate **2.5–2.9 mmol/l**	1. Approx deficit 400–500 mmol K
	2. Replace magnesium if low – see hypomagnesaemia protocol
	3. Replace K by mouth if able to take orally and if GI tract functions normally
	4. If not then give IV – see below
	5. Give around 100–120 mmol K per day orally as Sando K 3 tabs three times daily (108 mmol K)
	6. Monitor K daily until serum K >2.9 mmol/l then manage as above
Severe **<2.5 mmol/l or** **dysrhythmia**	1. Approx deficit 500–600 mmol
	2. IV potassium likely to be required
	3. Use preprepared bags of 500 ml saline 0.9 % or dextrose 5 % containing 20 or 40 mmol K
	4. 10 mmol/h is safe to give through peripheral vein
	5. 20 mmol/h can be given through large peripheral vein with ECG monitoring
	6. 40 mmol/h occasionally required for life threatening dysrhythmia or paralysis – can be given through central vein with ECG monitoring
Potassium **replacement**	1. Slow K 8 mmol per tablet – but note can ulcerate oesophagus and small intestine so avoid if dysphagia or intestinal motility impaired
	2. Sando K 12 mmol per tab – dissolves in water, unpleasant taste, safer but more expensive than Slow K
Potassium **preservation**	1. K sparing diuretics – Amiloride (better tolerated) and Spironolactone
	2. ACEI/ARB – inhibit aldosterone release

Appendix 3 Treatment of Hypocalcaemia

Severity	Action
Mild hypocalcaemia >1.9 mmol/L and asymptomatic	1. Give oral calcium supplements e.g. Sandocal 1000 2 tabs bd (Sandocal 1000 contains 25 mmol calcium)
	2. If post-thyroidectomy and serum calcium remains 1.9–2.1 mmol/l after 24 h increase Sandocal 1000 to 3 tabs bd
	3. If remains 1.9–2.1 mmol/l after 72 h despite Sandocal add alfacalcidol 0.25 μg od and repeat serum calcium at 1 week
Severe hypocalcaemia <1.9 mmol/L and/ or symptomatic	1. This is a medical emergency
	2. Give calcium gluconate 10 % 10 ml IV in 50–100 ml dextrose 5 % over 10 min with cardiac monitoring (contains 2.32 mmol calcium)
	3. Follow with calcium gluconate 10 % 100 ml (10 vials) in saline 0.9 % or dextrose 5 % infused at 50–100 ml/h to achieve normocalcaemia (contains 23.2 mmol calcium)
	4. Avoid calcium chloride which is more potent than calcium gluconate and causes tissue necrosis if extravasates
	5. If post-op hypocalcaemia following parathyroidectomy or thyroidectomy, give alfacalcidol starting at 0.25–0.5 μg od
	6. It is usually possible to treat the hypocalcaemia of renal failure with alfacalcidol alone – see Chap. 28
Treat the underlying cause	1. If hypomagnesaemia, give 20 mmol Mg as 10 ml of 50 % magnesium sulphate. Dilute to 50 ml in dextrose 5 % for central administration or to 250–500 ml in dextrose 5 % for peripheral administration. Infuse over minimum of 5 h, max 24 h
	2. If vitamin D deficiency, load with 3,200 iu cholecalciferol e.g. Fultium D3 4×800 iu capsules per day for 12 weeks, followed by maintenance dose of 800–1,600 iu cholecalciferol as Fultium D3 1–2 capsules per day indefinitely

Appendix 4 Treatment of Hypercalcaemia

Severity	Action
Serum calcium <3 mmol/l	1. Usually asymptomatic and does not require urgent correction
	2. Avoid factors that can aggravate hypercalcemia, including thiazide diuretic and lithium therapy, volume depletion, prolonged bed rest or inactivity, and a high calcium diet (>25 mmol or 1,000 mg/day)
Serum calcium 3–3.5 mmol/l	1. May be well tolerated if has risen slowly, if symptomatic then prompt treatment usually indicated
	2. Rehydrate then give IV biphosphonate
Serum calcium >3.5 mmol/l or symptomatic	1. Requires urgent treatment because risk of shock, coma, renal failure
	2. Rehydrate then give IV biphosphonate
	3. May need to consider dialysis if severe renal failure
Rehydration	1. Rehydrate with IV saline 0.9 % 3–4 l in first 24 h and 2–3 l daily thereafter aiming for urine output urine output >2 l/day
	2. IV fluid lowers serum Ca, but will not restore normocalcaemia
	3. Loop diuretics do not promote calciuresis but may be needed if develops fluid overload
	4. Be more cautious in elderly with renal impairment and with LV dysfunction
After rehydration – IV biphosphonates	1. IV biphosphonates are most beneficial for hypercalcaemia of malignancy but can still be used in other causes of hypercalcaemia
	2. Do not use until patients are rehydrated
	3. If GFR >30 ml/min and still hypercalcaemic after hydration, give IV zoledronate 4 mg over 15 min in 100 ml saline 0.9 %
	4. If GFR <30 ml/min after hydration give pamidronate according to the corrected serum calcium as follows: calcium <3.0 mmol/l: 30 mg; calcium 3–3.5 mmol/l: 60 mg; calcium >3.5 mmol/l: 90 mg
	5. Add pamidronate to saline 0.9 % at a concentration not exceeding 60 mg/250 ml and infuse at a rate not greater than 20 mg/h
	6. Full effect of IV biphosphonate may take 3–7 days with duration of action 1–2 weeks
Maintenance therapy	1. Discuss treatment options with relevant consultant
	2. Counsel patients contemplating long term maintenance with bisphosphonates re osteonecrosis of the jaw and a dental check before treatment
	3. IV zolendronate is preferred maintenance for myeloma and SC denosumab for breast cancer
	4. Oral clodronate sometimes still used for myeloma if cannot tolerate IV zolendronate or if patient choice because reduced risk osteonecrosis

Appendix 5 Treatment of Hypophosphataemia and Hypomagnesaemia

Severity of ↓ PO$_4$	Action
Mild **0.6–0.7 mmol/l**	No treatment required
Moderate **0.3–0.59 mmol/l**	1. Give Phosphate-Sandoz 1–2 tablets orally tds (each tab contains 16 mmol PO$_4$, 3 mmol K and 20 mmol Na) and repeat phosphate the following day
	2. Diarrhoea is a common side effect of oral phosphate therapy – risk can be reduced if given in at least 120 ml of water
	3. Review dose daily according to phosphate levels and stop when serum PO$_4$ >0.6 mmol/l
	4. If nil by mouth or symptomatic, give Addiphos 10–20 ml IV as below
Severe <0.3 mmol/l	1. Normal renal function – 20 ml Addiphos IV (20 ml vial contains 40 mmol phosphate, 30 mmol potassium and 30 mmol sodium) diluted in 500 ml of 0.9 % Saline or 5 % dextrose given over at least 4 h with repeat serum K, Ca and PO$_4$ 4 h after end of infusion
	2. Impaired renal function – 10 ml Addiphos IV given as above
	3. Side effects of IV phosphate include hypocalcaemia due to binding with calcium and AKI due to Ca-PO$_4$ precipitation in kidneys
	4. Usually safe to switch to oral phosphate when serum PO$_4$ >0.5 mmol/l

Severity of ↓ Mg	Action
Serum magnesium 0.4–0.6 mmol/l and asymptomatic	1. If patient eating then try oral magnesium glycerophosphate (4 mmol per tablet) aiming for an intake of 12–24 mmol/day
	2. Reduce dose if diarrhoea occurs and halve dose if renal impairment
	3. May require IV replacement if NBM or develops diarrhoea
	4. Monitor Mg, Ca and K daily
Serum magnesium <0.4 mmol/l OR symptomatic	1. IV Mg best given slowly as at high infusion rates a high proportion of infused Mg will be excreted via the kidneys
	2. Give 20 mmol Mg as 10 ml of 50 % magnesium sulphate. Dilute to 50 ml in glucose 5 % for central administration or to 250–500 ml in glucose 5 % for peripheral administration. Infuse over minimum of 5 h, max 24 h. Note conversion 1 g Mg=4 mmol Mg
	3. IV Mg may be required for up to 5 days, depending on deficit
	4. Halve dose if renal impairment
	5. Monitor Mg, Ca and K daily
Other indications for IV magnesium	1. Recurrent VT, torsade de pointes, status asthma
	2. Give 8 mmol IV bolus then check serum Mg and follow with 20 mmol over 24 h if <0.7 mmol/l

Appendix 6 Plasma Exchange

Each unit will have protocols for plasma exchange. Ours are based on the advice given in UpToDate and are reproduced below.

Indications for Plasma Exchange

These are renal, haematological and neurological. Renal indications are Goodpasture's syndrome and rapidly progressive renal failure due to ANCA positive vasculitis. The haematological indications are hyperviscosity syndrome usually in association with multiple myeloma, HUS-TTP and cryoglobulinaemia. Plasma exchange is also indicated for patients with severe Guillain-Barre syndrome, chronic inflammatory demyelinating polyneuropathy not responding to conventional therapy, and severe myasthenia gravis.

Plasma Exchange for ANCA Positive Vasculitis

1. Total number of exchanges – 7 on alternate days over a fortnight.
2. Plasma volume to be exchanged – 60 ml/kg
3. Replacement fluid – usually human albumin solution unless recent biopsy, in which case use albumin followed by FFP in ratio 3:1. If actively bleeding e.g. pulmonary haemorrhage or visible haematuria post biopsy we use FFP for all replacement fluid
4. If the patient requires haemodialysis – do the dialysis first

Plasma Exchange for Goodpasture's Syndrome

1. Total number of exchanges – Daily or alternate days for 2–3 weeks with serial assessment of clinical status and anti-GBM titres. If haemoptysis persists or anti-GBM titres remain positive we continue plasma exchange until haemoptysis resolves and anti-GBM titers become markedly suppressed or negative
2. Plasma volume to be exchanged – 4 litres
3. Replacement fluid – usually human albumin solution unless recent biopsy, in which case use albumin followed by FFP in ratio 3:1. If actively bleeding e.g. pulmonary haemorrhage or visible haematuria post biopsy we use FFP for all replacement fluid.
4. If the patient requires haemodialysis – do the dialysis first.

Plasma Exchange for HUS-TTP

1. Total number of exchanges – daily until the platelet count and the LDH (marker of haemolysis) are normal.
2. Plasma volume to be exchanged – 60 ml/kg.
3. Replacement fluid – Octaplas (a form of fresh frozen plasma that has been treated to reduce the risk of blood borne viruses in patients who are receiving very large volumes of FFP).
4. If the patient requires haemodialysis – do the dialysis first.

Hypocalcaemia

1. Plasma calcium commonly falls with citrate based anticoagulants (used in FFP) but also with human serum albumin. Calcium is bound to albumin in the circulation; therefore if you remove the albumin you will remove considerable quantities of calcium too.
2. If post PEX (Plasma Exchange) calcium <2.0 mmol/l, infuse 20 ml calcium gluconate 10 % (containing 4.4 mmol calcium) per session. This can be given during or after the session.

Hypofibrinogenaemia

1. Plasma fibrinogen commonly falls during plasma exchange. FFP contains modest quantities of fibrinogen which is the slowest clotting factor to be replenished. Daily exchanges in particular may cause significant hypofibrinogenaemia and risk of bleeding.
2. Do full clotting screen before each PEX (Plasma Exchange) and treat as follows:
   - Fibrinogen 1.0–1.5 g/l: best to defer PEX (Plasma Exchange) for a day if possible. Use FFP as replacement fluid for next exchange.
   - Fibrinogen <1.0 g/l: discuss with haematology. Postpone plasma exchange until the next day. Use FFP as replacement fluid for next exchange and consider giving one pool of cryoprecipitate (which contains fibrinogen) immediately after PEX (Plasma Exchange).

Hypotension

1. Stop ACEI as these drugs can cause hypotension during plasma exchange.

Appendix 7 Vasculitis Protocol

We use the European Vasculitis Study Group protocol for treatment of ANCA associated systemic vasculitis, summarised as follows:

Cyclophosphamide (CYC) – Pulsed Induction Protocol
1. IV pulses 15 mg/kg at 0, 2, 4, 7, 10, 13, 16, 19, 22 and 25 weeks (10 pulses in all).
2. Can give oral pulses 5 mg/kg for 3 days from 7 weeks if preferred.
3. Dose of CYC should be reduced if age >60 years or serum creatinine >300 μmol/l.
4. Max CYC pulse is 1,200 mg. Round dose down to nearest 50 mg.
5. Rx granisetron 2 mg orally before each pulse and domperidone 20 mg qds for 3 days after each pulse.
6. If WCC on day of pulse <4,000 cells/μL then postpone pulse until >4,000 cells/μL, checking WCC weekly. Reduce dose of pulse by 25 %.
7. Check WCC 10–14 days after pulse. If <3,000 cells/μL then reduce next pulse by 20 %. If <2,000 cells/μL reduce next pulse by 40 %.
8. Commonly give CYC with MESNA to protect against haemorrhagic cystitis. Use same dose as CYC – 20 % IV at start of treatment then 40 % orally at 4 and 8 h.
9. Usually continue CYC every 3 weeks until 3 months after remission achieved or until a lifetime maximum of 36 g has been given.

Prednisolone
1. Start at 60 mg daily for 1 week then reduce to 45 mg daily for 1 week, 30 mg daily for 1 week, 25 mg daily for 3 weeks, 20 mg daily for 2 weeks, 15 mg daily for 4 weeks, with view to reducing to 12.5 mg daily after 12 weeks and to 10 mg daily after 20 weeks (end of month 5).
2. Further reduction in steroid dose should be to 7.5 mg daily during months 12–15 and to 5 mg daily during months 15–18.
3. Flexibility in prednisolone dose±12.5 % allowed in the first 12 weeks and±25 % thereafter.

Azathioprine (AZA) – Remission Maintenance Dose
1. Switch CYC to AZA 3 months after remission achieved.
2. Dose of AZA should be 2 mg/kg, rounded down to nearest 25 mg.
3. Reduce dose by 25 % if age >60 years and by 50 % if age >75 years.
4. Check FBC and transaminases twice weekly for 1st month then every month for 5 months then every 2 months.
5. Withhold AZA if WCC <4,000 cclls/μL and postpone next dose until >4,000 cells/μL, checking WCC weekly. Reduce dose by 25 %.
6. If leucopenia severe (WCC <1,000 cells/μL) or prolonged (<4,000 cells/μL for >2 weeks) then restart AZA at 50 mg daily, increasing to target dose if weekly WCC permit.

Prophylaxis
1. Gastric protection – ranitidine or omeprazole for 6 months.
2. Fungal protection – nystatin 1 ml qds for 3 months.
3. Pneumocystis protection – avoid unless strong local preference in which case use septrin 480 mg three times per week for 3 months.
4. Bone protection – Adcal D3 2 tablets daily or equivalent if >50 years.
5. Cardiovascular protection – consider aspirin and statins, stop smoking.

Side Effects of Immunosuppressive Drugs

1. CYC – leucopenia, infection (usually respiratory and urinary), infertility, cancers, haemorrhagic cystitis, alopecia and amenorrhoea.
2. Steroids – osteoporosis, candidiasis (oral and vaginal), other infections, weight gain, diabetes, hypertension, cushingoid appearance, peptic ulcer, skin atrophy, cataract, fulminant VZV in susceptible subjects.
3. AZA – nausea, leucopenia, thrombocytopenia, infection, cancer, alopecia, cholestasis. Important interaction with allopurinol leading to severe leucopenia.

Further Reading

1. European Vasculitis Study Group protocol for treatment of ANCA associated Systemic Vasculitis. www.vasculitis.nl/media/documents/cyclops.pdf

Appendix 8 Glucose Lowering Drugs and CKD

Drug	Mode of action	Clearance	Relevant points	Use in CKD
Biguanide e.g. Metformin	Increases glucose uptake by tissues	Renal	Accumulates, risk of metformin induced lactic acidosis	Stop when eGFR <30 ml/min
Sulphonylurea e.g. Gliclazide	Stimulates insulin release	Renal	Accumulates, risk of hypoglycaemia	Reduce dose if hypoglycaemia a problem
Thiazoledinedione e.g. Pioglitazone	Increases the action of insulin	Hepatic	Risk of fluid retention, anaemia and bone fractures	No dose adjustment necessary but side effects may limit use in CKD
Glucagon-like peptide 1 (GLP1) analogue e.g. Exenatide	Stimulates insulin secretion, inhibits glucagon release, delays gastric emptying, increases feeling of fullness	Renal	Given subcut, can cause nausea	Avoid if eGFR <30 ml/min
Dipeptidyl peptidase-4 (DPP-4) inhibitor e.g. Linagliptin, Sitagliptin, Saxaglipitin, Vildagliptin	Inhibits the enzyme that breaks down GLP1	Renal except linagliptin	Linagliptin may cause troublesome cough and sore throat	No dose adjustment required for linagliptin; reduce dose of sitagliptin, saxagliptin, vildagliptin when eGFR <50 ml/min

Further Reading

1. National Kidney Foundation. KDOQI clinical practice guidelines for diabetes and Chronic Kidney Disease, 2012 update. Am J Kidney Dis. 2012;60:850–86.

Appendix 9 Dietary Potassium Advice

Most fruit and vegetables, milk and coffee are rich in potassium and should be limited or avoided by dialysis patients. More detailed advice is shown in the table below.

	High potassium (to limit or avoid)	Lower potassium alternatives
Drinks	Fruit and vegetable juices	All fizzy drinks, cordials and squashes,
	Coffee – up to 1 cup per day	Tea, fruit tea
	Milk or milky drinks – up to ½ pint/day	Spirits
	Malted drinks (Ovaltine/Horlicks), drinking chocolate	
	Beer, cider, lager, sherry, wine	
Fruit	All dried fruit	Apples or pears
	Bananas, mango, grapes, apricots, rhubarb, fresh grapefruit, pineapple, strawberries and avocado	Tinned fruit (drained of juice) Limit to maximum 3 portions daily
Vegetables	Tomatoes, beetroot, plantain, mushrooms, sweetcorn, aubergine, parsnip, spinach	All boiled vegetables, onion, carrot, turnip, cabbage, cauliflower, lettuce, cucumber, celery
Sweets	Chocolate, fudge, toffee, liquorice, black treacle	Boiled sweets, mints, fruit pastels, chewing gum, jam, honey, syrup
Snacks	All nuts	Snacks made from wheat, corn or rice (e.g. Doritos, Wotsits, Skips)
	All potato crisps	Popcorn
	Bombay mix	
Potatoes and alternatives	Baked or roast potatoes, chips	Boiled potatoes Rice, pasta, noodles, bread

Appendix 10 Dietary Phosphate Advice

Dairy products tend to be rich in phosphate and may require to be limited or avoided in dialysis patients. More detailed dietary phosphate advice is shown in the table below.

	Higher phosphate foods to reduce	Lower phosphate food alternative choices
Dairy	Milk	Soya milk
	Cheese incl. cheese sauce	Cottage cheese, feta, ricotta, parmesan, cream cheese
	Yoghurt	Double cream, whipping cream
	Eggs	Soya yoghurt
	Condensed and evaporated milk, dried milk, milk puddings, ice cream	Egg whites
Meat	Liver, kidney, liver and chicken pate, game birds	Beef, lamb, pork, turkey, rabbit, chicken
Fish	Mussels, scallops, sprats, whitebait, kippers, smoked fish, cod roe, herring roe	White fish e.g. haddock, plaice, halibut, sole, skate
		Oily fish e.g. tuna, trout, salmon
		Fish fingers, fish cakes, tinned crab, squid
		(once a week only – pilchards, sardines, prawns, herring or mackerel)
Breakfast cereal	All Bran, Bran Buds, Farmhouse Bran, muesli or cereals containing nuts or chocolate	All other cereals
Biscuits/cakes	Rye crispbread, oatcakes, flap jacks, scones, potato scones, fully coated chocolate biscuits	Cream crackers, water biscuits, digestives, rich tea, shortcake, crumpet, pancake, cream biscuits, wafers, Jaffa cakes, shortbread, Danish pastries, doughnut, half coated plain chocolate biscuits
Miscellaneous	Nuts, peanut butter, baking powder, marzipan, milk chocolate, cocoa, malted milk drinks, drinking chocolate, beer and ale	Plain chocolate or filled chocolates
		Gravy browning, Bisto
		Boiled sweets, chewy fruit sweets, jelly sweets, pastilles, peppermints, chewing gum, marshmallows, sherbet sweets

Appendix 11 Antibiotics for Urinary Tract Infection

Hospitals have region specific antibiotic protocols to control antibiotic resistance and emergence of antibiotic associated infection. The table below gives an example of appropriate antibiotic prescribing for urosepsis. Please refer to local guidance.

Indication and typical duration	1st line	2nd line/alternative
Lower UTI		
Uncomplicated UTI: Treatment duration 3 days women, 7 days men	Trimethoprim PO 200 mg bd or Nitrofurantoin PO 50–100 mg qds	
Pregnancy: Treatment duration 7 days	Avoid trimethoprim 1st trimester and nitrofurantoin 3rd trimester	
Complicated UTI e.g. elderly with confusion or febrile	Add stat dose of Gentamicin IV and reassess	
Acute pyelonephritis		
Treatment duration 7–14 days depending on severity	Amoxicillin IV 1 G tds + Gentamicin IV Step down to Co-amoxiclav PO 375–625 mg tds	Allergy: Ciprofloxacin IV 400 mg bd + Gentamicin IV. Step down to Ciprofloxacin PO 500–750 mg bd
Pregnancy: Treatment duration 14 days	Co-amoxiclav PO 375–625 mg tds	If penicillin allergy seek advice from microbiologist
Urinary catheter sepsis		
Change catheter after 24–48 h of treatment Treatment duration 5 days guided by clinical response Treatment duration 14 days if gram negative septicaemia	Amoxicillin IV 1 G tds + Gentamicin IV Step down to Co-amoxiclav PO 375–625 mg tds	Allergy: Ciprofloxacin IV 400 mg bd + Gentamicin IV. Step down to Ciprofloxacin PO 500–750 mg bd
Acute prostatitis/epidymo-orchitis		
Treatment duration 14 days 4 weeks treatment may prevent chronic infection	Ciprofloxacin PO 500 mg bd	

Notes
Nitrofurantoin can only be used for cystitis as absorption is poor and blood levels are inadequate to treat pyelonephritis. Anorexia, nausea, vomiting and diarrhoea are common side effects. Nitrofurantoin can cause hepatitis so check liver function tests in symptomatic patients. This is particularly important if used long term in prophylaxis. Nitrofurantoin should be avoided if eGFR less than 60 ml/min partly because it will be ineffective as result of inadequate urine concentration and partly because it can cause painful peripheral neuropathy.

    Trimethoprim can cause a transient rise in serum creatinine by inhibiting tubular secretion of creatinine. This may be relevant in some cases where moderate rise in creatinine would have implications on management e.g. a renal transplant recipient. Importantly, it can also cause hyperkalaemia by mimicking amiloride-like effects on the distal tubule. It is best avoided in those with CKD, particularly if they have a tendency towards hyperkalaemia e.g. because of acidosis or ACE inhibitor use.

Appendix 12 Iron and Erythropoeisis Stimulating Agents

Iron and ESA therapy have transformed the management of renal anaemia. There remains some controversy regarding doses and targets. Our current practice is outlined below.

Oral or intravenous iron? Iron should be given orally in the first instance for predialysis or PD patients. Ferrous fumarate 305 mg bd is a suitable oral preparation. IV iron is recommended for HD patients and for predialysis and PD patients in whom oral iron is not tolerated or ineffective

Intravenous iron preparations

Drug	Brand	Notes
Iron saccharate	Venofer	Bolus injection. Most suited to use in HD
Iron isomaltose	Monofer	Licensed for total dose infusions, therefore suited to out-patient use
Iron dextran	Cosmofer	Also licensed for total dose infusions. Cheaper, but takes longer to infuse than iron isomaltose (4–6 h vs. 30 min)

IV iron loading dose for predialysis and PD patients – this is best achieved by total dose infusion using iron isomaltose. A single dose of up to 20 mg/kg can be prescribed although in practice we usually give a maximum of 1G at a time. This is done by adding the drug to 100 ml 0.9 % saline and infusing over 30 min. No test dose is required.

IV iron loading dose haemodialysis – Iron saccharate is usually given through the machine during haemodialysis. A typical prescription might be 100 mg three times a week as a bolus injection over 5 min to a total of 1G (10 doses). A test dose of 20 mg in 1 ml over 1–2 min is required.

Maintenance iron – the need for maintenance intravenous iron after a loading dose is dictated by the haemoglobin response and the serum ferritin. We measure serum ferritin monthly on haemodialysis and at least 3 monthly in predialysis and PD patients, aiming for a level somewhere between 200 and 800 ng/ml (the optimal level is not yet known). Predialysis and PD patients may be able to maintain their iron stores with oral iron if tolerated.

IV iron adverse reactions –Transient hypotension can occur if intravenous iron is give too quickly. Parenteral iron can also cause allergic reactions which may occasionally be life threatening though the risk of anaphylaxis is much lower than it was with earlier preparations.

ESA preparations

Drug	Brand	Notes
Epoetin alfa	Eprex	Dose given 2–3 times/week
Epoetin beta	Neorecormon	Dose given 2–3 times/week
Darbepoeitin	Aranesp	Initial dose: once weekly if HD, fortnightly for predialysis and PD
		Dose may be given once monthly once target achieved

ESA starting doses – The recommended starting dose for Aranesp is 0.45 mcg/kg IV or SC as a weekly injection (usually 30 mcg) or 0.75 mcg/kg once every 2 weeks (usually 50 mcg) if this is preferred. Many units will have an ESA delivery service for their home patients, most of whom are taught to self-administer subcutaneously.

Maintenance ESA – KDIGO suggest an upper limit for Hb of 115 g/l in adults with CKD, while recognising that some patients may have improvements in quality of life at Hb >115 g/l and will be prepared to accept the risks provided that ESAs are not used intentionally to increase Hb >130 g/l.

It may take a few weeks before the impact of dose changes of Aranesp are seen in achieved Hb, and for this reason frequent dose changing is not recommended. Hb should be checked fortnightly or monthly initially then, once stable, every 3 months.

Further Reading

1. Kidney Disease: Improving Global Outcomes (KDIGO) Anaemia Work Group. KDIGO Clinical Practice Guideline for Anaemia in Chronic Kidney Disease. Kidney inter., Suppl. 2012;2:279–335.

Appendix 13 Phosphate Binders

We take a number of factors into account when choosing a phosphate binder, principally the serum calcium and the presence or absence of vascular calcification.

Calcium acetate – We give calcium acetate (Phosex) unless the serum calcium is greater than 2.45 mmol/l or patient already has vascular calcification. The main side effect is hypercalcaemia which limits its usefulness. A usual starting dose is 1 g (one tablet) before lunch and 2 g (2 tablets) before the evening meal, unless the patient's main meal is lunch. The dose can be increased if necessary and if tolerated but providing the serum calcium does not exceed 2.5 mmol/l.

Calcium carbonate – Calcium carbonate (Calcichew) is an orange flavoured tablet that the patient must chew immediately before food. Some like the taste and some do not. It contains more calcium than Phosex, which is a reason to try Phosex first. The usual starting dose of Calcichew is 500 mg (one tablet) chewed before lunch and 500 mg (one tablet) chewed before the evening meal. Hypercalcaemia is the main side effect. Calcichew only works in an acid environment which means it is not effective in patients who take ranitidine (H2 antagonist) or omeprazole (proton pump inhibitor). The dose can be increased if necessary and if tolerated, as per Phosex above.

Aluminium Hydroxide – Aluminium hydroxide (Alucaps) is the most effective of the phosphate binders. The main side effect is high serum aluminium, the risks of which include dialysis dementia, EPO resistant anaemia and vitamin D resistant bone disease. The starting dose is 2 capsules twice daily before food. If Alucaps are prescribed then we advise checking the serum aluminium monthly to ensure that this does not exceed 1 nmol/l.

Sevelemar – The main attraction of Sevelemar (Renagel, Renvela) is that it contains neither calcium nor aluminium. Unfortunately it is expensive and not particularly well tolerated with many patients complaining of gastrointestinal side effects. Renagel comes as 400 or 800 mg tablets while Renvela is either an 800 mg tablet or sachet. Three 800 mg tablets/sachets three times daily are required for Sevelemar to be maximally effective, and not everyone can manage this. We tend to start with a low dose and then work up gradually.

Lanthanum – Lanthanum (Fosrenol) is another non-calcium non-aluminium binder. It is effective and well tolerated if given with or after food but causes nausea and vomiting if taken before. Recommended starting dose is one 500 mg tablet chewed or crushed with or immediately after food three times daily. This can be titrated with 750 or 1,000 mg tablets every 2–3 weeks towards a total daily dose of 3,000 mg daily if necessary and if tolerated. Lanthanum is a useful phosphate binder in patients whose baseline serum calcium is greater than 2.45 mmol/l and in those who already have vascular calcification.

Drug	Brand	Notes
Calcium acetate	Phosex	Calcium containing phosphate binders
Calcium carbonate	Calcichew	
Aluminium hydroxide	Alucaps	Aluminium containing phosphate binder
Sevelemar hydrochloride	Renagel	Non-calcium, non-aluminium containing phosphate binders
Sevelemar carbonate	Renvela	
Lanthanum	Fosrenol	Another non-calcium, non-aluminium containing phosphate binder

Appendix 14 Control of Calcium After Parathyroidectomy

Most units will have a protocol describing how to manage calcium at the time of parathyroidectomy. We describe ours below.

Indications for Parathyroidectomy
Prolonged stimulation of the parathyroid glands in dialysis patients may eventually cause the glands to secrete PTH autonomously, a condition known as tertiary hyperparathyroidism, and when this happens parathyroidectomy may be required.

Control of Hypocalcaemia After Surgery
Hypocalcaemia is extremely common post-op as calcium is sucked from the blood back into the bones when it is no longer under the influence of PTH (so-called hungry bone syndrome). This is more likely to occur when the serum ALP is raised.

Pre-op
1. Give alfacalcidol 2–4 μg daily for 3–5 days pre-op and continue post-op until calcium is normal. This is safe for 3 days even if calcium is high pre-op.
2. Continue cinacalcet until admitted for surgery and then stop.
3. Continue usual phosphate binders pre- and perioperatively.
4. Remember to check calcium and phosphate pre-operatively.

Post-op
1. Check calcium within 1 h of surgery and then every 4–6 h, depending on serum calcium, until advised otherwise. If normal at 48 h then further trouble is very unlikely.
2. If calcium falls below normal but remains greater than 1.9, give oral calcium supplements unless symptomatic (see below). Give Sandocal 1,000 effervescent tablets (25 mmol calcium per tablet) 2 tablets three times daily as starting dose, between meals to improve absorption.
3. If calcium <1.9 mmol/l, or if symptomatic, give IV calcium gluconate 10 % 30 ml (containing 6.9 mmol calcium) over 10 min. NB extravasation of calcium can cause tissue necrosis – for this reason calcium gluconate is preferred to calcium chloride which contains 3 × more calcium
4. Follow this with 100 ml calcium gluconate 10 % added to 150 ml dextrose 5 % and infused at 20–40 ml/h (2–4 mmol/h).
5. Continue alfacalcidol but keep doubling the dose to a maximum of 8–10 μg per day if substantial calcium supplements are required.
6. Always check Mg once daily while hypocalcaemic and replace if necessary. Hypomagnesaemia inhibits the release of PTH which effectively means that the serum calcium will not correct until the serum Mg has been corrected.

After Discharge
1. Check calcium two to three times per week until stable.
2. Sandocal can usually be decreased fairly quickly, but may have to be continued for up to 2 weeks especially if serum ALP was high pre-operatively.
3. Alfacalcidol can generally be decreased to 2 μg per day after about a week.
4. Some patients will require maintenance therapy with alfacalcidol 1–2 μg daily, if their parathyroid remnant fails to function.

Symptoms of Hypocalcaemia
1. Any one or a combination of the following may suggest hypocalcaemia: numbness, paraesthesia, muscle weakness, abdominal cramping. Check for Trousseau's phenomenon (spasm of hand muscles provoked by pressure on the nerves supplying the muscles) when measuring blood pressure post-op.

Appendix 15 Prescribing for Chronic Pain in CKD

Analgesics

Paracetamol	eGFR	Dose	Notes
	>60 ml/min	1 g every 6 h	Reduce dose in those ≤50 kg regardless of renal function
	30–60 ml/min	Maximum 4 g daily	
	15–30 ml/min		
	<15 ml/min	Maximum 3 g daily	
NSAIDs	>60 ml/min	No dose adjustment	Best avoided when eGFR <60 ml/min
	30–60 ml/min	Caution	
	15–30 ml/min	Avoid	
	<15 ml/min	Avoid	
Codeine	>60 ml/min	30–60 mg every 6 h	Best avoided in CKD 5 and on dialysis
	30–60 ml/min	Dose as above	
	15–30 ml/min	30 mg every 6 h	
	<15 ml/min	Avoid if possible	
Tramadol	>60 ml/min	Max 100 mg every 6 h	Use cautiously in CKD 4/5
	30–60 ml/min	Dose as above	
	15–30 ml/min	50–100 mg every 8 h	
	<15 ml/min	Max 50 mg twice daily	
Oral morphine	>60 ml/min	No dose adjustment	Best avoided in CKD 4/5. Could try 2.5–5 mg cautiously
	30–60 ml/min	75 % of usual dose	
	15–30 ml/min	Avoid if possible	
	<15 ml/min	Avoid if possible	
Transdermal fentanyl	>60 ml/min	No dose adjustment	Use 12 mcg/h patch as initial dose in CKD5 and on dialysis
	30–60 ml/min	As above	
	15–30 ml/min	75 % of usual dose	
	<15 ml/min	50 % of usual dose	
Subcutaneous alfentanil	>60 ml/min	100–500 µg as bolus dose	Possible role in acute pain on dialysis
	30–60 ml/min	As above	
	15–30 ml/min	As above	
	<15 ml/min	As above	

Anti-emetics

Metoclopramide	eGFR	Dose	Notes
	>60 ml/min	10 mg every 8 h	Higher risk of dyskinesia in CKD 5
	30–60 ml/min	As above	
	15–30 ml/min	As above	
	<15 ml/min	5 mg every 8 h	
Haloperidol	>60 ml/min	1–2.5 mg orally every 6 h	May cause hypotension and sedation
	30–60 ml/min	As above	
	15–30 ml/min	As above	
	<15 ml/min	0.5 mg orally every 8 h	
Cyclizine	>60 ml/min	25–50 mg three times daily	Risk of hypotension and arrhythmias in CKD 5 and on dialysis
	30–60 ml/min	As above	
	15–30 ml/min	As above	
	<15 ml/min	Avoid	
Ondansetron	>60 ml/min	4–8 mg up to three times daily	Regular use can cause constipation. May help renal itch
	30–60 ml/min	As above	
	15–30 ml/min	As above	
	<15 ml/min	As above	

Adjuvants

Amitriptyline	eGFR	Dose	Notes
	>60 ml/min	No dose adjustment	Slow titration in CKD to minimise anticholinergic side effects
	30–60 ml/min	As above	
	15–30 ml/min	As above	
	<15 ml/min)	As above	
Carbamazepine	>60 ml/min	No dose adjustment	
	30–60 ml/min	As above	
	15–30 ml/min	As above	
	<15 ml/min	As above	
Valproate	>60 ml/min	No dose adjustment	
	30–60 ml/min	As above	
	15–30 ml/min	As above	
	<15 ml/min)	As above	
Gabapentin	>60 ml/min	No dose adjustment	Significantly lower doses used in CKD and on dialysis
	30–60 ml/min	300 mg at night	
	15–30 ml/min	300 mg alternate days	
	<15 ml/min)	300 mg post dialysis	

Further Reading

1. The Renal Drug Handbook, Caroline Ashley and Aileen Dunleavey. 4th ed. 2014. Radcliffe Publishing Ltd.

Appendix 16 Optimal Medical Care on Haemodialysis

Health domains	Action and goals
Renal Health	1. Fluid balance – aim for weight gain between dialysis sessions of not more than 2 kg
	2. Potassium – pre-dialysis potassium <6.0 mmol/l
	3. Acid base balance – pre-dialysis bicarbonate >24 mmol/l
	4. Renal bone disease – pre-dialysis phosphate less than 1.1–1.7 mmol/l with corrected calcium in normal range for your hospital and PTH two to nine times the upper limit of normal (see section on renal bone disease)
	5. Anaemia – haemoglobin 100–115 g/l with or without EPO and iron (see section on anaemia)
Vascular Health	1. Vascular risk factors – these include diet, exercise, smoking, blood pressure and cholesterol
	2. Blood pressure – post-dialysis blood pressure <133–155/70–90 mmHg with or without antihypertensive drugs (see section on blood pressure control)
	3. Lipid lowering is controversial. The latest KDIGO guidelines recommend not starting statins in adults on haemodialysis but continuing them if patients are already receiving these drugs
	4. Regular reviews of eyes and feet in patients with diabetes
Psychosocial Health	1. Holidays – holiday dialysis can be arranged both in the UK and abroad but plans need to be made several months in advance
	2. Psychological – dialysis patients may become anxious or depressed
	3. Social support – some dialysis patients are completely independent, while many will rely on carers. The areas to be covered here include washing, dressing, housework, meals and shopping
General Health	1. Immunisations – ensure yearly influenza and pneumococcal vaccine every 5 years
	2. Nutrition – aiming for good appetite, not losing weight and serum albumin >36 g/L
Review of Treatment Modality	1. Assessment for transplantation where appropriate – a transplant will improve survival and quality of life for most patients under the age of 75
	2. Consider dialysis withdrawal where appropriate – when it becomes clear that dialysis in prolonging a patients suffering rather than giving them any quality of life

Appendix 17 Immediate Management of PD Peritonitis

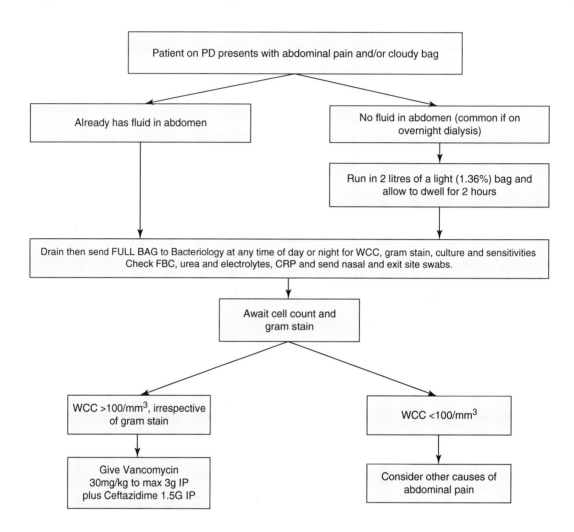

Antibiotics can be added to 2 litres of Physioneal or Extraneal PD fluid. In practice we usually use a light bag (1.36 % glucose) of Physioneal. Dwell time should be minimum of 6 h up to a maximum of 12 h. APD patients do not need to convert to CAPD unless peritonitis is severe enough to require admission.

Appendix 18 Urokinase Protocol for Blocked Tunnelled Lines

You may be called to the dialysis unit because a patient's tunnelled line has blocked. The following protocol is based on a letter in NDT by Shavit and colleagues (*NDT* 2007;22:666). There are three steps, as follows:

Urokinase protocol	
Step 1	Add 7 ml saline to 25,000 unit vial of urokinase. Lock each lumen with 2.5 ml for 10 min, followed by 0.5 ml push down each lumen 5 min later and a further 0.5 ml push down each lumen 5 min after that. Leave for another 5 min then re-aspirate and flush with saline
Step 2	For catheters with poor flow (150–200 ml/min) infuse 125,000 units urokinase in 50 ml normal saline throughout treatment using three way tap via heparin line. Normal heparin dose to continue throughout treatment
Step 3	For catheters with persisting low flow (200–250 ml/min and step 2 has been used on 3 consecutive treatments) infuse 125,000 units urokinase in 50 ml normal saline simultaneously through each catheter lumen (total dose 250,000 units urokinase) over 90 min. Haemodialysis should be restarted immediately afterwards, initially with a blood pump speed of 250 ml/min increasing to 300 ml/min if possible
Contraindications to urokinase	
Step 1	No contraindications
Step 2 + 3	Previous haemorrhagic stroke at any time, non-haemorrhagic stroke within 1 month, active bleeding from a non-compatible site, known brain tumour, INR greater than 3, major surgery or trauma within 3 weeks, bleeding DU within 3 weeks, pregnancy, non-compressible vascular puncture

Need for Consent

No consent is required for a urokinase lock. Patients should however provide written consent for a urokinase infusion in step 2 and step 3. The evidence we have is that this dose is 14 times less than the dose given to lyse clot in patients with pulmonary embolus. Only one bleeding complication was reported in a series of 19 infusions reported by Shavit and colleagues in NDT, and this was on a patient who was also taking aspirin and warfarin. Under the circumstances we feel that the risks of urokinase infusion are probably less than the risks of catheter replacement in a patient with a blocked or poorly functioning tunnelled line.

Index